Great Medical Discoveries

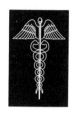

Insulin

by Janice M. Yuwiler

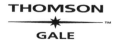

LUCENT BOOKS

An imprint of Thomson Gale, a part of The Thomson Corporation

THOMSON

GALE

Detroit • New York • San Francisco • San Diego • New Haven, Conn. • Waterville, Maine • London • Munich

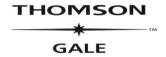

For Itz Schreibman (1924–2005), who despite battling diabetes
for seventy-five years lead a full and productive life.

LIBRARY OF CONGRESS CATALOGING-IN-PUBLICATION DATA

Yuwiler, Janice.
  Insulin / by Janice M. Yuwiler.
    p. cm. — (Great medical discoveries)
  Includes bibliographical references and index.
  ISBN 1-56006-930-9 (hard cover : alk. paper)
  1. Insulin—Juvenile literature. 2. Diabetes—Juvenile literature. I. Title. II. Series.
QP572.I5Y89 2005
616.4'62—dc22   2004023516

CONTENTS

FOREWORD

Throughout history, people have struggled to understand and conquer the diseases and physical ailments that plague us. Once in a while, a discovery has changed the course of medicine and sometimes, the course of history itself. The stories of these discoveries have many elements in common—accidental findings, sudden insights, human dedication, and most of all, powerful results. Many illnesses that in the past were essentially a death warrant for their sufferers are today curable or even virtually extinct. And exciting new directions in medicine promise a future in which the building blocks of human life itself—the genes—may be manipulated and altered to restore health or to prevent disease from occurring in the first place.

It has been said that an insight is simply a rearrangement of already-known facts, and as often as not, these great medical discoveries have resulted partly from a reexamination of earlier efforts in light of new knowledge. Nineteenth-century monk Gregor Mendel experimented with pea plants for years, quietly unlocking the mysteries of genetics. However, the importance of his findings went unnoticed until three separate scientists, studying cell division with a newly improved invention called a microscope, rediscovered his work decades after his death. French doctor Jean-Antoine Villemin's experiments with rabbits proved that tuberculosis was contagious, but his conclusions were politely ignored by the medical community until another doctor, Robert Koch of Germany, discovered the exact culprit—the tubercle bacillus germ—years later.

Accident, too, has played a part in some medical discoveries. Because the tuberculosis germ does not stain with dye as easily as other bacteria, Koch was able to see it only after he had let a treated slide sit far longer than he intended. An unwanted speck of mold led Englishman Alexander Fleming to recognize the bacteria-killing qualities of the penicillium fungi, ushering in the era of antibiotic "miracle drugs."

That researchers sometimes benefited from fortuitous accidents does not mean that they were bumbling amateurs who relied solely on luck. They were dedicated scientists whose work created the conditions under which such lucky events could occur; many sacrificed years of their lives to observation and experimentation. Sometimes the price they paid was higher. Rene Launnec, who invented the stethoscope to help him study the effects of tuberculosis, himself succumbed to the disease.

And humanity has benefited from these scientists' efforts. The formerly terrifying disease of smallpox has been eliminated from the face of the earth—the only case of the complete conquest of a once deadly disease. Tuberculosis, perhaps the oldest disease known to humans and certainly one of its most prolific killers, has been essentially wiped out in some parts of the world. Genetically engineered insulin is a godsend to countless diabetics who are allergic to the animal insulin that has traditionally been used to help them.

Despite such triumphs there are few unequivocal success stories in the history of great medical discoveries. New strains of tuberculosis are proving to be resistant to the antibiotics originally developed to treat them, raising the specter of a resurgence of the disease that has killed 2 billion people over the course of human history. But medical research continues on numerous fronts and will no doubt lead to still undreamed-of advancements in the future.

Each volume in the Great Medical Discoveries series tells the story of one great medical breakthrough—the first gropings for understanding, the pieces that came together and how, and the immediate and longer-term results. Part science and part social history, the series explains some of the key findings that have shaped modern medicine and relieved untold human suffering. Numerous primary and secondary source quotations enhance the text and bring to life all the drama of scientific discovery. Sidebars highlight personalities and convey personal stories. The series also discusses the future of each medical discovery—a future in which vaccines may guard against AIDS, gene therapy may eliminate cancer, and other as-yet unimagined treatments may become commonplace.

INTRODUCTION

Diabetes and the Miracle of Insulin

Diabetes, a deadly disease, is recorded in the medical records of many peoples, beginning with the Egyptians in 1500 B.C. Diabetes occurs when a person's body loses the ability to use glucose, a sugar formed during digestion and the major source of energy for the body. Instead of being taken into the cells and used for energy, glucose builds up in the blood, causing damage to many parts of the body.

Prior to the discovery of the hormone called insulin, diabetes was a death sentence. In the 1800s, a child diagnosed with diabetes could expect to live less than a year and a half after symptoms of the disease appeared. The survival rate for an adult diagnosed with diabetes at age thirty was longer, at slightly more than four years. But the life left to live was not pretty. Infections and complications typically killed patients diagnosed with diabetes as adults. For children and severe diabetics, coma and death came quicker. Diabetes destroyed the body, and the wasting away could be terrible. One patient was described as follows: "When he came to the hospital he was emaciated, weak and dejected; his thirst unquenchable; and his skin dry, hard and harsh to the touch, like rough parchment."[1]

Type 1 Diabetes

Experts now realize that there are at least two types of diabetes. Five to 10 percent of all diabetic patients have type 1 diabetes. Although scientists do not completely understand the process, it appears that people with type 1 diabetes have an autoimmune reaction to the cells in the pancreas that make insulin. In other words, the person's immune system perceives the insulin-producing cells as invaders and proceeds to attack and destroy them. As a result, the body loses its ability to produce insulin. Without insulin, glucose cannot enter the cells to nourish them. To stay alive, people with type 1 diabetes must continuously resupply their bodies with insulin. Usually this means taking injections of insulin several times a day.

Typical Features of Type 1 Diabetes

Age of Onset	Under forty years old; most common in childhood
Body Weight	Thin to normal weight
Type of Onset	Fairly rapid, with symptoms appearing and worsening over weeks to months
Treatment	Must take insulin, usually several times a day
Blood Sugar Levels	Up and down; hard to keep in the normal range
Family History	Typically, no known family history
Risk Factors	Increased risk if strong family history of type 1 diabetes; slightly increased risk if one other family member has type 1 diabetes
Cause	Genetic predisposition and exposure to an environmental trigger that causes an autoimmune response that destroys the insulin-producing beta cells in the pancreas
Test Results	Blood sugar usually high; glycosylated hemoglobin levels high; islet cell antibodies or insulin autoantibodies present

Type 2 Diabetes

Not all people with diabetes depend on injections of insulin to stay alive. More than 90 percent of people with diabetes in the United States have type 2 diabetes. In type 2 diabetes, the body has become resistant to the effects of insulin. Either the pancreas produces too little insulin to move glucose into the cells, or the cells do not recognize insulin properly.

The typical person with type 2 diabetes is over forty years old, overweight, and has a family history of diabetes. However, with the increase in overweight and inactive youth, more young people than ever are developing type 2 diabetes. Again, scientists are not certain of the cause, but it appears that the muscle cells of overweight people are less responsive to insulin. In addition, an obese person's pancreas must produce large amounts of insulin to service all the cells, and it may be that the pancreas becomes exhausted over time. The chance of developing type 2 diabetes increases with age and weight gain, especially among people who get little or no exercise.

Extent of the Problem

As many as 18 million Americans suffer from diabetes, but over 5 million do not know they have the disease. Untreated, diabetes is fatal, causing serious damage to many parts of the body, such as the eyes, kidneys, blood vessels, nerves, feet, and legs. Diabetes is a major risk factor for heart disease and stroke and is the leading cause of blindness, kidney failure, and amputations in the United States today.

The cost of diabetes is staggering. In the United States, the cost was an estimated $132 billion in 2003. Almost 70 percent of that amount was spent directly on health care. Costs related to disability, loss of productive work, and early death accounted for the remaining 30 percent. And the problem is growing: Approximately 1.3 million new cases of diabetes are diagnosed each year.

The Miracle of Insulin

The discovery of insulin in 1922 by Frederick Banting and Charles H. Best, along with John James Rickard Macleod and James Bertram Collip, was heralded as a miracle. By taking insulin, people with diabetes could again process their food and live normal lives. Dr. Frank N. Allan was in medical school when insulin was discovered. Looking back fifty years later, he emphasized the importance of insulin: "The one factor of predominant importance in the management of diabetes is still insulin. In the crises of diabetic management, there is no substitute. After fifty years nothing can take its place. It has . . . restored health and protected the lives of persons who would otherwise have little hope of survival."[2]

In 1922 Charles H. Best (left) and Frederick Banting (right) discovered the hormone insulin, a discovery that has saved the lives of countless diabetics.

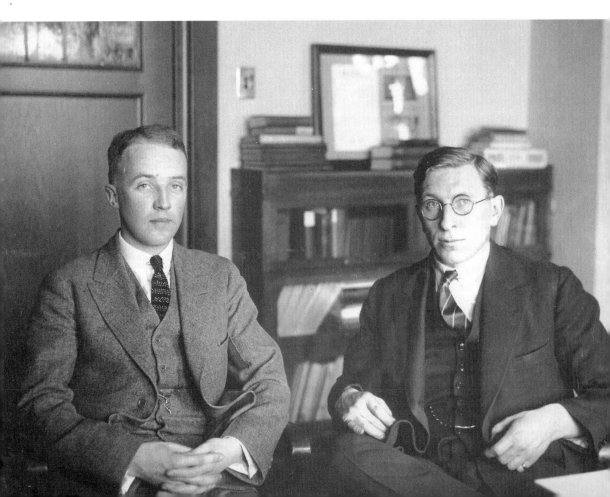

Typical Features of Type 2 Diabetes

Age of Onset	Over forty years old; most common in older adults, although growing more common in overweight and inactive young people
Body Weight	Overweight; occasionally occurs in people of normal weight
Type of Onset	Slow onset, with symptoms appearing gradually over months or years; classic symptoms may not be present
Treatment	May be able to control with diet and exercise or oral medication; may need to take insulin
Blood Sugar Levels	Without the ups and downs of type 1 diabetes, usually easier to control
Family History	Typically, others with type 2 diabetes in the family
Risk Factors	Increased risk if person is overweight and inactive, if there is a strong history of type 2 diabetes in the family, if person had gestational diabetes during pregnancy, or if person is of Native American, African American, Hispanic, or Japanese American descent
Cause	Not well understood but appears to be combination of genetics, lifestyle, insulin resistance, and insufficient production of insulin by beta cells
Test Results	Blood sugar can be very high but usually only moderately high; glycosylated hemoglobin levels mildly or moderately high; islet cell antibodies or insulin autoantibodies not present

Although insulin has saved the lives of millions of people with diabetes, it is not a cure. A social worker in the mid-1930s wrote: "With the discovery of insulin in 1922 came the hope, not only for added years of life, but also for happiness and normality in those added years. For these benefits there was a definite price to pay which to most diabetic patients must have seemed small, the regular use of insulin and care in choosing the diet." Still, she wondered if "the inescapable injections of insulin and constant weighing and selecting of food seem[ed] a terrific responsibility, and did the constant attention demanded prevent them from living as they formerly had lived."[3]

People with diabetes must continually measure the glucose in their blood, adjusting their medications and their diets to keep their blood sugar within normal levels. If they do not, they risk blindness, loss of limbs, kidney failure, stroke, heart attack, and death. New technologies continually make it easier to monitor blood sugar level, inject insulin, and live more flexible lives, but there is still no cure for diabetes. Advances in surgery, genetic engineering, and antibody therapy are offering new hope that a cure for diabetes will soon be found.

CHAPTER 1

Treating the Sugar Sickness

Diabetes is an ancient disease, and a deadly one. For thousands of years people could describe its symptoms but had no success in treating the disease. Even when researchers linked the disease to the body's inability to use sugar, solving the problem proved difficult.

People with diabetes cannot process sugars from the food they eat. Normally food is broken down by the intestines into several compounds, including glucose, the main sugar required by the body. With the hormone insulin acting as a key to open cell membranes, glucose in the blood enters the cells and is used for energy.

About half of the glucose produced from a meal is stockpiled in the liver in a form called glycogen to be used when the level of glucose, the blood sugar, in the blood drops too low. The remainder of the glucose not used by the cells is stored in the muscles or converted to fat for long-term storage. The normal body has a system of checks and balances that constantly measures blood sugar. If there is too much sugar, the pancreas produces more insulin to move glucose into the cells. If there is too little, glycogen from the liver is released or the body converts fat to glucose for the cells' use.

People with diabetes either lack insulin or their cell membranes do not recognize and accept the insulin they produce. For these people, the body's system of checks and balances does not work, and glucose, prevented from entering the cells, builds up in their blood. The kidneys try to remove the excess glucose from the blood and wastewater, but the volume of sugar is too great. Sugar spills into the patient's urine, creating two of the earliest recognized symptoms of diabetes: sugar in the urine (glycosuria) and excessive urination.

History

Excessive urination was first mentioned in the ancient Egyptian document of medical knowledge, the Ebers Papyrus. The Ebers Papyrus, written around 1500 B.C., describes a disease in which people produce an enormous quantity of urine. By 400–200 B.C., physicians in India had also noticed the sweetness of the urine produced by people with diabetes. The Charaka Samhita, one of the oldest and most important ancient writings on ayurvedic medicine, describes "a feeling of sweetness in the mouth, burning sensations in the hands and feet, and of a urine so sweet that it attracted the ants."[4]

By A.D. 229, the Chinese and Japanese had noted that "the urine of diabetics was very large in amount and was so sweet, that it attracted dogs."[5] In fact, one of the techniques used to diagnose diabetes was to taste a patient's urine. If it was sweet, the person had what some called the sugar sickness.

Hindu medical writings of the sixth century refer to diabetes as *Madhumeha*, or "honey urine." Today's term, *diabetes*, is the name given the disease by Aretaeus of Cappadocia, a famous Greek physician of the first century. Aretaeus believed diabetes drained patients of more liquid than they could consume. In his words, "Diabetes is a wasting of the flesh and limbs into urine. . . . The patient never [ceases] to make water and the discharge is . . . incessant. . . . The patient does not survive long for the marasmus [wasting] is rapid and death speedy. The thirst is ungovernable, the copious potations [frequent drinks] are more than equaled by the profuse urinary discharge."[6]

A Sixth-Century Hindu Description of Diabetes

Physician Joseph H. Barach, in his article "Historical Facts in Diabetes," quoted from Hindu medical writings of the sixth century that refer to diabetes as Madhumeha, or "honey urine," describing:

a disease of the rich and one that is brought about by gluttonous over-indulgence in rice, flour and sugar. This order of the disease is ushered in by the appearance of morbid secretions about the teeth, ears, nose and eyes. The hands and feet are very hot and burning, and the surface of the skin is shining as if oil had been applied to it. This is accompanied by thirst, and a sweet taste in the mouth. The different varieties of this disease are distinguished from each other by the symptoms of deranged humors, and by the colour of the urine.

If the disease is produced by phlegm, insects approach the urine, the person is languid, his body becomes fat, and there is a discharge of mucus from the nose and mouth, with dyspeptic symptoms and looseness of the skin. He is always sleepy, with cough, and difficult breathing.

Later, the Latin word *mellitus*, which means honey, was added to the name of the disease, which is now called diabetes mellitus.

Treatment

Early physicians were well aware diabetes was a deadly disease. Indian physicians in the sixth century noted, "All the hereditary and congenital forms of this disease are incurable; and if not properly treated, they generally terminate in sweet urine, which is incurable."[7] Yet for over three thousand years no one knew how to help victims of the disease.

Healers tried. Egyptians used a combination of ground earth, water, bones, wheat, and lead over a period of four days to treat diabetes. Precisely how the ingredients were combined and applied and what effect the treatment had remain a mystery. Only the ingredients are listed in the ancient writings that have survived to the present day.

Ancient Greek physicians prescribed exercise, preferably on horseback, as a cure for diabetes. They hoped moderate pressure on a patient's urethra would reduce

The eleventh-century Arab physician Avicenna was the foremost medical authority of his day, but even he knew of no effective treatment for diabetes.

the excessive urination. While modern medicine has shown exercise can help patients with type 2 diabetes, horseback riding would have produced few if any cures.

Over five hundred years after the Greeks, Avicenna, the great Arab physician, set forth to record the complete medical knowledge of his time. He was an outstanding clinician himself, but even with all his skill and the knowledge he collected, he knew of no effective treatment for diabetes.

By the nineteenth century, not much had changed. Physicians used the same methods to treat diabetes that they used for every other disease, with the same lack of success. By bleeding, cupping, or blistering patients, they tried to draw off whatever was causing the illness, but these means were ineffective.

Doping, the use of drugs to relieve symptoms, was also popular in the 1800s and continued into the twentieth century. In 1919 a leading U.S. diabetologist complained that the habit of using opium to dope diabetic patients "is very difficult to break even at the present time."[8] Although doping did nothing to treat or cure diabetes, opium seemed to reduce the despair of dying patients.

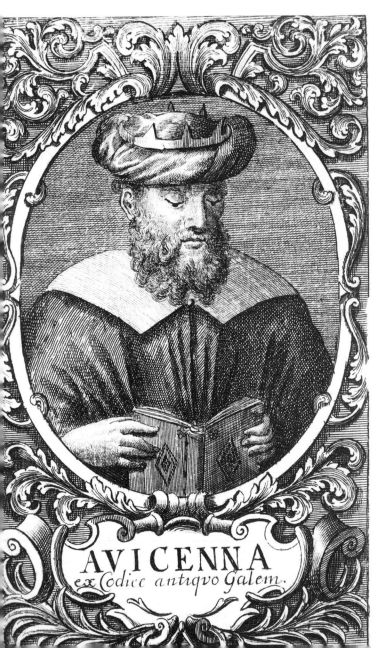

AVICENNA
ex Codice antiquo Galeni.

Avicenna (980–1037), "the Prince of Physicians"

The great Arab physician of his day, Avicenna influenced not only the practice of medicine in his own time but the practice of medicine for five centuries after his death. Among his many writings, he attempted to codify medical knowledge in a form similar to the medical encyclopedias of today. He believed that diabetes might have been primary or secondary to another disease and that it affected the liver. According to Dr. Joseph H. Barach, author of the article "Historical Facts in Diabetes":

Avicenna observed that diabetic patients have an irregular appetite, suffer great thirst, nervous exhaustion, an inability to work, and loss of sex function. . . . Translated from Avicenna's writings: The kidneys attract humors from the liver in greater quantities than they are able to retain. The urine leaves a residue like honey. Avicenna also observed that carbuncles and phtisis are frequent complications. He described diabetic gangrene, and finally, it was his opinion that treatment was not effective.

Addressing the Symptoms

Without knowing the cause of diabetes, healers could only treat symptoms of the disease. The most obvious symptom was excessive urination. A person with diabetes might pass as much as ten to fifteen quarts of urine a day. The loss of that much fluid left the person with unquenchable thirst, hunger, and fatigue. To compensate for the loss of fluid, and to build up a patient's strength, doctors fed their patients more food. This practice had the opposite of the desired result. Since people with diabetes cannot use sugars from the food they eat and symptoms are caused by sugar building up in the blood, overfeeding just made the problem worse.

In the late 1850s, Priorry, a French doctor, took the idea of overfeeding patients with diabetes one step further, with disastrous results. Priorry had his patients eat extra-large quantities of sugar, which only sped up the accumulation of excess sugar in the blood and added more stress to the body. In fact, a physiologist who advocated Priorry's ideas followed the diet when he developed diabetes himself, lapsed into a diabetic coma, and quickly died.

Symptoms of Diabetes

- Excessive thirst

- Frequent urination

- Extreme hunger

- Unusual weight loss

- Increased fatigue

- Irritability

- Blurred vision

Sometimes doctors did not even attempt to treat complications from the disease. For example, when uncontrolled, diabetes can damage blood vessels in the legs, reducing circulation. This means cuts or sores on the legs may not heal and can become severely infected or even gangrenous. Gangrene, or the death of tissue around an injury, can be fatal if the dead tissue is not removed. Doctors would often let such conditions run their course, knowing that surgical wounds might not heal and patients risked developing severe infections. Because diabetic patients were likely to die from complications of surgery, doctors saw little point in subjecting people already mortally ill to more agony.

Diet

Meanwhile, a few doctors were on the right track, although their work was often ignored. These doctors wondered if the excess sugar in the urine and blood of patients with diabetes was caused by the body's inability to process food for nourishment. If so, these doctors reasoned, overfeeding these patients to help them gain weight and strength might be doing more harm than good. Perhaps restricting the amount of food consumed could make a difference. In 1798 John Rollo, surgeon general for the British Royal Artillery, prescribed a reduced-calorie diet for one of his captains who had developed diabetes and kept the man alive for over a year. A second patient was unwilling to follow the diet and did not live as long as the captain had. Unfortunately, not much attention was paid to Rollo's efforts at the time. It would be several generations before other doctors realized that restricting the amount of food consumed could make a difference.

In the mid-1800s French physician Apollinaire Bouchardat began designing special diets as a way of treating diabetes. He advised his patients to use fresh fats instead of carbohydrates, to avoid milk because it contained the sugar lactose, and to avoid alcohol because of its sugar content. Bouchardat invented gluten bread and pushed the advantages of green vegetables. He experimented with periodic fasts and stressed the importance of a very low calorie diet. He also noticed that exercise increased his diabetic patients' tolerance for carbohydrates. Bouchardat is said to have told one patient who was begging for more food, "You shall earn your bread by the sweat of your brow."[9]

In 1870 and 1871 Bouchardat observed that sugar in the urine of his patients with diabetes disappeared when they ate less food. He noticed this when food rationing was imposed on Paris during the Franco-Prussian War. A huge leap forward had been made in the treatment of diabetes. People with diabetes could be kept alive longer if they ate less.

Low-Carbohydrate Diets

Carbohydrates seemed to be particularly hard for people with diabetes to digest. Thus, diets low in carbohydrates were prescribed for patients with diabetes. Under the assumption the problem was limited to carbohydrates, many doctors added heavy amounts of fat to the diet to make the diet more appealing and to help patients gain weight. Low-carbohydrate diets, even if they contain lots of fat, tend to be unappetizing over time. As a result, many patients had trouble sticking to their diets.

In 1902 Carl von Noorden in Germany announced an oat cure for diabetes. According to von Noorden, people with diabetes could eat carbohydrates as long as they were foods made from oatmeal. This offered relief from the low-carbohydrate diets. Nutritionists rushed to research why oats could be tolerated by people with diabetes when other carbohydrates could

Carbohydrate Metabolism

Carbohydrates are one of the components of food. They are found in grains, fruits, vegetables, dairy products, and sweets. The metabolism of carbohydrates begins with digestion, which breaks down food into components the cells of the body can use to grow, reproduce, and do the work of the body.

Digestion begins in the mouth when saliva mixes with food, starting the process of breaking down food into its components. The food and saliva mixture is passed by swallowing to the esophagus, a long, stretchy tube about ten inches long, that uses muscles along its length to push food to the stomach, where it is mixed with gastric juices that further break down the food. From the stomach, food passes to the small intestine. In the small intestine, with the help of the pancreas, liver, and gallbladder, the body finishes turning the food into nutrients that can be used by the cells. These nutrients pass from the small intestine into the bloodstream, which carries them to the cells. The remainder of the food that cannot be used by the body passes into the large intestine and colon, where the body absorbs water and any remaining minerals it can use. The leftover is pushed to the rectum, where it waits until it is pushed out of the body as waste.

The digestive system turns carbohydrates into three main types of sugars: glucose, fructose, and galactose, which are carried by the bloodstream to the cells. The presence of glucose in the blood causes the pancreas to produce the hormone insulin. Insulin binds to cell membranes and allows glucose to enter the cells, where it is used for energy. About half the glucose generated by a meal is stored as glycogen in the muscles and the liver to be used later. Between meals, the liver will release glucose into the system to nourish the cells when the supply of glucose in the blood decreases, for example, when someone exercises and the muscles need more food. The liver can also make glucose using the body's fat and protein stores.

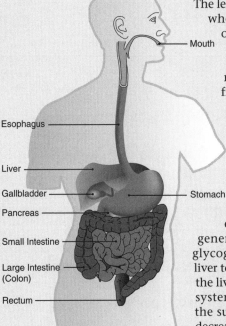

Mouth

Esophagus

Liver

Gallbladder

Pancreas

Small Intestine

Large Intestine
(Colon)

Rectum

Stomach

not. In fact, the oat cure was only the most popular of many fad diets offered to people with diabetes with varying success. Other proposed but ineffective cures included the milk diet, the rice cure, and potato therapy.

Not Just Carbohydrates

Dr. Frederick Allen, one of the leading diabetologists in the United States in the early twentieth century, was interested in which diets were most effective for his patients with diabetes. Through extensive research, Dr. Allen found that people with diabetes had trouble metabolizing not only carbohydrates but fats and proteins, too. All foods seemed to overburden the bodies of individuals with diabetes.

Dr. Allen believed that any of the diets that worked to reduce sugar in the urine worked only because the diet was low in calories. In fact, the high fat content of some of the low-carbohydrate diets may have accelerated diabetic comas in patients by causing buildup of half-metabolized fats called ketones.

Ketones can be smelled in the urine or on the breath of anyone who has an excess amount of them in the body. Rooms and hospital wards filled with patients dying of diabetes were instantly recognizable by the sickish-sweet, rotten-apple-like smell of ketones. In the late 1800s and early 1900s doctors knew that once they smelled ketones in a patient's urine, coma and death would soon follow. To prevent death, they tried to neutralize the half-metabolized fats by giving comatose patients a solution of baking soda. This treatment, however, rarely worked in the early stages of a diabetic coma and never worked in the later stages.

Undernutrition and Starvation Diets

The lack of success treating the later stages of diabetes was offset by the glimmer of hope seen with low-carbohydrate and low-calorie diets. People with milder cases of diabetes (type 2) who both exercised and restricted the amount of food they ate could eliminate sugar in their urine. However, they were not cured of the disease. If they went back to eating a normal diet, the symptoms of diabetes returned.

Most people who successfully controlled their disease were older and had type 2 diabetes. For children and people with severe or type 1 diabetes, the future was not as bright. Because the bodies of children and people with type 1 diabetes do not make enough insulin to handle even low-carbohydrate and low-calorie diets, these people needed a diet that bordered on starvation to stay alive. The amount of calories a person could eat was determined individually.

First the person fasted until the sugar disappeared from the urine. Then food was slowly introduced and the urine monitored for sugar. The daily calorie intake was set at the amount of food the person could eat before sugar spilled into the urine. If the person got an

The photo on the left shows a young girl in the 1920s on a starvation diet to treat her diabetes. On the right, the same girl is shown later, after being treated with insulin.

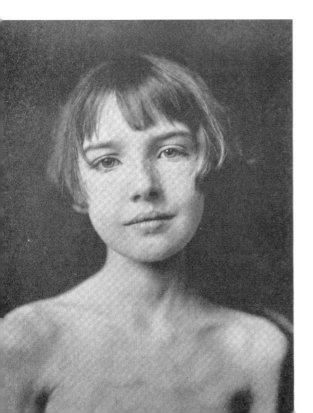
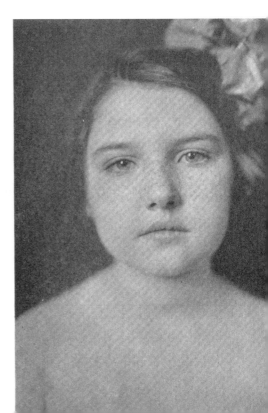

infection and the diabetes got worse, the diet would become even stricter.

Some doctors locked patients in their rooms to keep them from eating more. One young patient described the diet as a nightmare and hated the doctors who imposed it. Another cheated by eating toothpaste, birdseed, or whatever he could find. A nurse who worked on a diabetic ward in the early 1900s described the patients as having "big stomachs, skin-and-bone necks, skull-like faces, and feeble movements."[10]

Controversy

Asking weak diabetic patients to fast was highly controversial. These people had come to the hospital suffering from excessive thirst, hunger, and weight loss. Now they were being asked to fast until sugar disappeared from their urine. Patients' families would complain that their loved ones were too weak to fast. Patients who complained they were too hungry to fast were told that fasting would lessen their hunger. Weak, emaciated patients were told more exercise would help them use their food and build their strength. And when the method did not work, the number of calories in the diet was lowered further.

Dr. Allen defended the starvation diets, also called undernutrition, based on his research. He admitted such diets were hard to follow. He agreed they would not cure the disease and, at most, allowed people to live a bit longer. He acknowledged that people who were severely diabetic might die of starvation instead of diabetes. However, his research showed there was nothing else to do for a person whose body could not process food.

In general, Dr. Allen's diets were easier to tolerate than the low-carbohydrate diets because they were more balanced. People on Dr. Allen's diets tended to feel better because the natural hunger from dieting and fasting was easier to cope with than the hunger from high sugar levels. Even so, the diets were hard to follow and did not work for everyone. Some patients died of starvation, and those with severe diabetes deteriorated as quickly on the diets as they did without them.

Use of Undernutrition

Although starvation diets offered the best hope for people with diabetes, it is unclear how widely they were used. The treatment was accepted by medical schools and doctors who kept up to date with medical advances. However, there were other, less knowledgeable doctors who continued to drug or overfeed their patients. Those who sold patent medicines continued to promise that their products would cure diabetes. Others with diabetes turned to prayer, faith healing, and Christian Science.

Dr. Elliott P. Joslin did much to spread the therapy of undernutrition. Based in Boston, Dr. Joslin wrote many articles for physicians and patients, promoting undernutrition as a treatment for diabetes. Dr. Joslin described diabetes as the best of the chronic diseases, clean, not contagious, seldom unsightly, often painless, and unusually susceptible to treatment.

Whereas Dr. Allen was stern, forbidding, and a tireless scientist, Dr. Joslin was warm and charming, conveyed a sense of hope to his patients, and was particularly popular among children. Many children who were refused care elsewhere went to Boston to be treated by Dr. Joslin.

Dr. Joslin may have been deliberately overoptimistic to keep up the morale of his patients, as well as his own spirits. As leading diabetologists, Dr. Joslin and his friend Dr. Allen worked day in and day out with starving and dying patients. Both had little to offer their patients other than starvation. The need for a cure or better treatment was pressing.

CHAPTER 2

Searching for a Cure

The cause of diabetes eluded doctors and scientists for years. Aretaeus of Cappadocia thought diabetes was caused by diseases that attacked the bladder and kidneys or perhaps by the bite of a reptile. In the eleventh century, Avicenna, "the Prince of Physicians," thought diabetes might be caused by another disease or was perhaps even a disease of its own. He believed both the liver and the kidneys were affected by diabetes. Thomas Willis, an English physician at Oxford University in the seventeenth century, claimed diabetes was a blood disease because sugar appeared in the blood before it appeared in the urine. No one had yet discovered which organ of the body was involved.

Early Clues

The first clue about the role of the pancreas in diabetes dates to 1682. Johann Brunner, a Swiss physician, found that removing large portions of the pancreas caused excessive thirst and urination in animals, but he did not make the connection to diabetes or digestion. In 1788 Thomas Crawley suggested that diabetes might be caused by an injury to the pancreas. Crawley had performed an autopsy on a man who had died from diabetes and discovered his pancreas was damaged. Again, no one recognized the

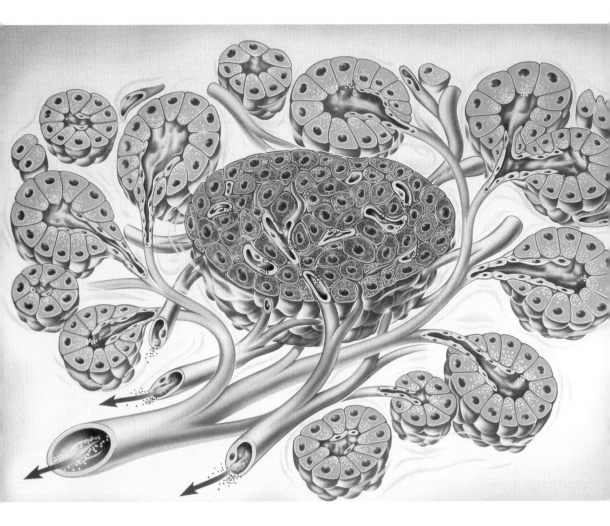

This drawing of pancreatic cells shows an islet of Langerhans (center) surrounded by acinar cells. The discovery of these cells brought researchers closer to understanding the role of the pancreas in diabetes.

significance of these findings, and the clues they provided to the role of the pancreas in digestion and diabetes were ignored.

In the early 1800s the French physiologist Claude Bernard was able to link diabetes to the process the body uses to convert food to sugars that nourish the body. That is, he realized that diabetes is linked to digestion, a major conceptual breakthrough. Bernard's research showed that the liver stores glycogen and secretes a sugary substance into the bloodstream that the body uses for energy. He reasoned that diabetes must be caused by the liver releasing too much sugar into the blood. The liver was the wrong organ, but Bernard was such a dominant figure in physiology and medicine in Europe that his theory went largely unquestioned for decades.

In 1869 Paul Langerhans, a German medical student, described two systems of cells in the pancreas: acinar cells, which secrete digestive juices via ducts into the small intestine; and small clusters, or little islands, of ductless cells. The clusters or islets seemed to float in a sea of acinar cells, but Langerhans could not determine their function. A few scientists took notice. The French histology expert Gustave Edouard Laguesse named the ductless cells the islets of Langerhans. Laguesse went on to propose that the islets performed some function besides secreting digestive juices. Twenty years later a chance occurrence cemented the role of the pancreas in diabetes.

In 1889, at the University of Strassburg, Germany, Joseph von Mehring, a physician, was studying digestion. He was curious about the role of the pancreas and wondered what would happen if he removed a dog's pancreas. Although he thought such a surgery would be impossible, his colleague Oskar Minkowski volunteered to perform the surgery. The next day a laboratory assistant complained he could not keep the dog's cage clean. Even though the dog was house-trained, the dog was urinating all over his cage. Minkowski, remembering the symptoms of diabetes, immediately tested the dog's urine. Sure enough, there was sugar in the urine. By removing the pancreas, Minkowski had caused diabetes. This time the world took notice.

Role of the Pancreas

Was it the lack of pancreatic juices that caused diabetes? Many researchers tried cutting or blocking the ducts that led from the pancreas to the intestine. These experiments stopped the flow of pancreatic secretions, causing some trouble with digestion, but symptoms of diabetes did not appear. In 1893 the French researcher Hédon removed the majority of a dog's pancreas and placed a tiny portion under the dog's skin, blocking connections between the pancreas and the digestive system. The dog recovered and showed no signs of diabetes. When Hédon removed the tiny bit of pancreas, the dog developed diabetes. It seemed the pancreas had two functions: helping with digestion and helping the body use sugar.

Scientists had known for years about external secretions, including the pancreatic juices, that pass through ducts into the small intestine. At the time, scientists were just discovering that ductless glands, such as the thyroid, ovaries, and pituitary, secrete hormones directly into the bloodstream. Given the results of their experiments, scientists guessed the islets of Langerhans might be ductless glands producing a hormone that helped the body use sugar.

In 1901 Eugene Opie at Johns Hopkins University confirmed this guess. Although he did not find evidence of the hormone itself, Opie proved there was a connection between diabetes and the islets of Langerhans. Pancreases from people who had died from diabetes had damaged islets of Langerhans.

The link between the pancreas and diabetes, especially the link to the islets of Langerhans, gave physicians an idea. Since doctors were having success treating thyroid disease with extracts of the thyroid, it seemed possible diabetes could be treated with extracts of the pancreas. Soon more research was being devoted to the islets of Langerhans and the pancreas than any other organ of the body. However, extracting a substance from the pancreas proved to be more difficult than anyone expected. Over four hundred researchers and physicians tried, but for almost three decades no one was able to extract a substance from the pancreas that could treat people with diabetes.

The Pancreas

The pancreas is a soft, spongy organ shaped like a banana. One end is thick, and the other end trails off into a small tail. It is located behind the stomach at the level of the navel. The pancreas produces several substances that are key to the body's ability to digest and use food. These substances are produced by different types of cells. The acinar cells produce digestive juices that flow through ducts from the pancreas into the small intestine and help convert food into components that can be used by cells throughout the body. Scattered throughout the acinar cells, like small islands, are clusters of a different type of cell. These clusters are called the islets of Langerhans. There are no ducts leading from the islets. Instead, cells within the islets produce hormones that are important in the use of sugar by the body for energy. The islets actually include three types of cells: alpha, beta, and delta cells. All three cells produce hormones that regulate the body's use of sugar. The beta cells store and produce the hormone insulin. The presence of glucose in the blood triggers the beta cells to deliver more or less insulin to the bloodstream as needed to maintain the amount of glucose within a certain range.

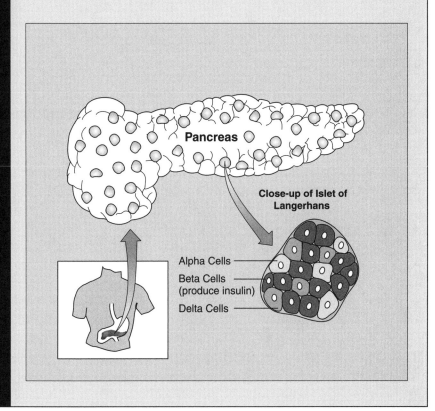

Pancreas

Close-up of Islet of Langerhans

Alpha Cells
Beta Cells (produce insulin)
Delta Cells

How Insulin Works

As shown in Carol Lewis's article "Diabetes: A Growing Public Health Concern," insulin acts like a key to open the door of the cell and allow glucose to enter. In fact, insulin binds to a receptor in the cell membrane, changing the shape of the membrane in such a way that glucose can enter and be used by the cell for energy. Without insulin, glucose cannot enter the cell, because the structure of the cell's membrane prevents glucose from entering. Glucose backs up in the blood of people with type 1 diabetes because there is no insulin to bind to the cell's receptor and let the glucose in. For people with type 2 diabetes, either there is something wrong with the receptor site that will not allow insulin to bind properly and open the cell wall, or there is not enough insulin available to bind to the cells and let glucose enter.

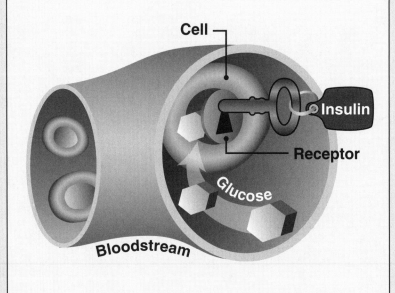

Like a key unlocking a door, insulin opens cell receptors so that glucose can enter the body's cells and be used for energy.

Georg Ludwig Zuelzer

In the early 1900s, Georg Ludwig Zuelzer, a young internist in Berlin, analyzed a number of pancreatic compounds and prepared concentrated versions of some of them, called extracts. Zuelzer—a persistent extractor—used alcohol to develop a pancreatic extract he called acomatrol. On June 21, 1906, Zuelzer injected acomatrol into a comatose fifty-year-old man with diabetes. The next day he gave the patient another injection of acomatrol. Miraculously, the patient seemed to come back from the edge of the grave. His overall condition improved, his appetite returned, and his severe dizziness disappeared. However, there was very little acomatrol available. When the extract ran out, the patient sank back into a deep coma and died on July 2, 1906. But Zuelzer was not discouraged. In his own words, "Whoever has seen how a patient lying in agony soon recovers from certain death and is restored to actual health will never forget it."[11]

Zuelzer had run out of acomatrol because supplies of pancreases were hard to obtain, the extract was difficult to make, and the extract would eventually lose its potency. Zuelzer approached the drug company Schering for help. Schering agreed to provide him with technical and financial support and filed for a patent on his work.

In the summer of 1907 Zuelzer again tried acomatrol on diabetic patients. The extract produced astounding results. It completely reversed the excessive urination and buildup of ketones in one patient and drastically reduced symptoms in others. However, a few of the patients did not seem to benefit. Worse, almost all the patients experienced vomiting, fever, and convulsions after the injections. Despite severe problems with the extract, Zuelzer was moved to proclaim, "It is possible through the injection of a pancreatic extract to eliminate the excretion of sugar, acetone, and acetoacetic acid by a diabetic without making any changes in the patient's diet."[12]

Good Canceled by Bad

J. Forschbach, a worker in the clinic directed by the famous Oskar Minkowski in Germany, obtained samples of Zuelzer's acomatrol and tried it on three dogs and three people with diabetes. The undesirable effects were so severe that Forschbach stopped the experiments, fearing he might do long-term damage. Forschbach noted, "It will be difficult to convince a patient who has been made severely ill by a single injection that this result was connected to a significant beneficial effect upon his diabetes."[13]

When a batch of acomatrol that had lost its potency caused no negative effects, Forschbach became convinced the active ingredient was the same ingredient that had caused the bad reactions. Forschbach's results were published in 1909 and reflected his belief that the active ingredient of the pancreatic extract was too toxic to be used. His findings were discouraging and dampened the building excitement about a pancreatic extract that would cure diabetes.

About the same time, Schering decided the results did not justify the costs and the drug company stopped funding Zuelzer. Zuelzer continued on as best he could, and in 1911 the Hoffman–La Roche chemical firm provided funding for Zuelzer to continue his work. There were still problems with the extract. One batch gave the test animals severe convulsions; another had no effect. Zuelzer was just getting ready for a new round of experiments with a promising new batch when World War I began. The hospital where Zuelzer worked was turned over to the military, and Zuelzer was sent to the front.

According to historian Michael Bliss, "The main effect of Zuelzer's work was probably to set back the search for an effective pancreatic extract. His published findings, plus Forschbach's report, seem to have convinced researchers of the impossibility of the enterprise: even if you did get an extract with anti-diabetic effects, whatever good effects it might have would be more than cancelled out by its bad effects."[14]

Ernest Lyman Scott

Ernest Lyman Scott was determined to find a safe pancreatic extract. A high school teacher studying advanced science through a correspondence course, Scott leapt at the chance to teach and study at the University of Chicago. He began work on his master's degree in 1909. Despite the lack of support from his adviser, he insisted on searching for a pancreatic extract that would cure diabetes, the disease that had killed one of his students.

From what he read and studied, Scott was convinced that the hormone scientists were searching for was a protein. He thought previous attempts had failed either because the powerful external pancreatic secretion destroyed the hormone or because exposure to air caused the hormone to oxidize. If he could get the pancreas to stop functioning, or atrophy, while leaving the islets of Langerhans intact, Scott thought he could make an extract of the islets without fear that the powerful pancreatic secretions would destroy the hormone. Lydia Dewitt, an American pathologist, had already tried something similar but had never tested her extract on living creatures.

Scott had little success at getting the pancreas to atrophy and finally gave up on the procedure. Instead, he tried two different methods to extract the hormone from the pancreas and prevent oxidation. Like Zuelzer before him, Scott made one extract using alcohol. For the other extract, he used slightly salty water and low heat. Scott had no success with the alcohol extract, but the water extract seemed to work: Three of the four diabetic dogs treated with the water-based extract showed improvement. The amount of sugar in their urine decreased, and in Scott's words, "if one dared say it, [the dogs] seemed even brighter for a time after the injection than before it."[15] Scott was convinced he had been successful. He wrote: "First, there is an internal secretion from the pancreas controlling the sugar metabolism. Second, by proper methods this secretion may be extracted and still retain its activity."[16]

Roadblocks

Anton Carlson, Scott's thesis adviser, was not convinced Scott had found a cure. Knowing the literature that questioned the effectiveness of pancreatic extracts, Carlson was concerned Scott had not controlled his experiments properly. Most likely concerned for the university's reputation, Carlson rewrote Scott's conclusions prior to the publication of his thesis in the *American Journal of Physiology*. In summarizing his work, Scott had stated injections of the pancreatic extract temporarily lowered the amount of sugar in the urine of diabetic dogs. To this statement, Carlson added, "It does not follow that these effects are due to the internal secretion of the pancreas in the extract."[17] Unsurprisingly, this disclaimer discouraged other researchers from studying or using Scott's methods; thus Scott's discovery was ignored for years. After all, in Scott's words, "Who would read the thing [Scott's thesis] when the author says it means nothing."[18]

Scott attempted to continue his work but never again had access to the laboratory facilities he needed. He approached several recognized experts with his results, including J.J.R. Macleod, who later played a major role in the discovery of insulin, but received no encouragement or assistance to continue his efforts. In the end, Scott was forced to drop his work on the pancreatic extract to study problems relating to blood sugar and earn a living to support his family.

Israel Kleiner

A few years after Scott's work was published, Israel Kleiner, a young American, became interested in blood sugar and pancreatic extracts while working with S.J. Meltzer at the Rockefeller Institute in New York. Together they were testing how fast research animals with and without diabetes processed injections of sugar. They found the injected sugar was rapidly processed by animals without diabetes, but in diabetic animals, the sugar continued to circulate in the blood. However, if a solution of pancreatic tissue was injected along with the sugar, the diabetic animals processed the sugar with almost the same speed as nondiabetic animals. Intrigued, Kleiner and Meltzer began experiments to see how pancreatic extracts would affect the ability to process sugar in diabetic dogs. They reported promising results in 1915, but their work ground to a halt when their funding was diverted because of World War I.

Ernest Lyman Scott (left) and Israel Kleiner researched the effects of pancreatic tissue extracts on dogs.

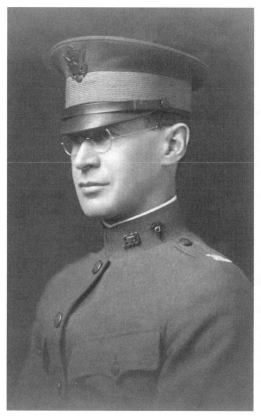
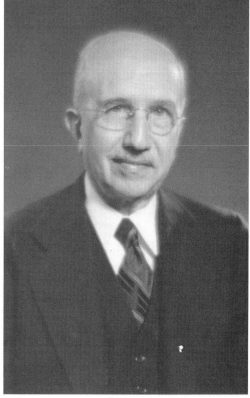

After the war, Kleiner took up where they had left off. With the aid of a new, more efficient way of testing blood sugar, he began testing a new pancreatic extract. Afraid that any chemicals used to extract compounds from the pancreas might themselves cause a change in blood sugar, Kleiner used only slightly salted distilled water to prepare the extracts. In carefully controlled experiments, Kleiner measured the blood sugar of diabetic dogs before and after the extract was injected into the dogs' veins. In every one of the sixteen experiments, the pancreatic extract caused the dog's blood sugar to fall rapidly, sometimes by as much as 50 percent.

Kleiner ran control experiments to be sure his results were not caused by something other than the extract, for example, the injected liquid diluting the blood. He made extracts of other types of tissues to see if he would obtain the same drop in blood sugar as with pancreatic tissue, but he never did.

Kleiner wrote up his findings in relation to what was known in the field. He reported only one problem: a

Measuring Sugar Levels

For a long time the only way to test the success or failure of treatments for diabetes was to measure the amount of sugar in a patient's urine. Although the urine sugar test is not as accurate as the blood sugar test, early blood sugar tests required as much as fifty milliliters, or roughly ten teaspoons, of blood. It was impossible to test blood sugar frequently when so much blood was needed for each test. Instead, researchers calculated the ratio of the sugar dextrose (D) to nitrogen (N) in the urine. This D/N ratio was considered a better measurement than the amount of sugar in the urine alone, and scientists usually used both measurements to support their conclusions.

As laboratory techniques improved, testing procedures requiring less blood were developed. This made testing the impact of pancreatic extracts easier and gave the later researchers an advantage. For example, in 1911 E.L. Scott was unable to measure blood sugar because the amount of blood required was too large. A decade later, Nicolas Paulesco analyzed blood sugars using a method that required twenty-five milliliters, or five teaspoons, of blood. In 1921 Charles Best used a method that required 0.2 milliliters of blood, or less than one-twentieth of a teaspoon.

mild fever that sometimes was associated with injection of the extract. Since this effect was not particularly severe, Kleiner concluded his experiments might be the foundation for an extract that could be used for patients with diabetes. Despite his impressive work and compelling results, Kleiner left the Rockefeller Institute in 1919 for a university that did not have the resources to support major animal research and did none of the follow-up work he had recommended.

Nicolas Paulesco

At the Romanian School of Medicine in Bucharest, Nicolas Paulesco, a distinguished professor of physiology, was also experimenting with extracts of the pancreas. Paulesco had been working on the problem since his student days in Paris in the 1890s, but his work had been interrupted by the Austrian occupation of Bucharest and the post–World War I turmoil in Romania.

Like Kleiner and Scott, Paulesco prepared his pancreatic extract using slightly salty distilled water. He then looked at the impact his pancreatic extract had not only on blood sugar in diabetic dogs, but also on sugar in the urine and the presence of ketones. Paulesco reported spectacular decreases in blood sugar, along with reductions in glycosuria (sugar in the urine) and ketones.

Like Kleiner, Paulesco ran control experiments to check for factors other than the pancreatic extract that might have caused the spectacular decreases he observed. Paulesco also tested the effect of extracts made from other organs of the body. Since his extract often caused fever, Paulesco even induced fever in his experimental animals to be sure fever by itself did not reduce blood sugar or glycosuria.

Paulesco did not conduct as many experiments as Kleiner did, and he did not tie them as thoroughly to the existing literature and knowledge of the day. Nonetheless, his experiments were more varied than anyone else's to date, his results were good, and he was committed to solving problems with his extract. The results of his work were published between 1920 and 1921 and held promise of a future cure for the thousands of people with diabetes who were struggling to stay alive on starvation diets.

CHAPTER 3

The Summer and Fall of 1921

Frederick Banting and Charles H. Best are known as the discoverers of insulin. Like others before them, their attempts to obtain a pancreatic extract were accompanied by both success and failure. In the end, their work at the University of Toronto in the summer and fall of 1921 proved that a pancreatic extract, later named insulin, could save the lives of people with diabetes.

According to Frederick Banting, it all began the evening of October 31, 1920. Banting, a surgeon, spent the evening preparing a lecture on carbohydrate metabolism for medical students at Western University in Ontario, Canada. When he finished, he picked up the November issue of the journal *Surgery, Gynecology and Obstetrics* and read Moses Barron's article "The Relation of the Islets of Langerhans to Diabetes with Special Reference to Cases of Pancreatic Lithiasis." As Banting later said,

> It was one of those nights when I was disturbed and could not sleep. I thought about the lecture and about the article and . . . finally about two in the morning after the lecture and the article had been chasing each other through my mind for some time, the idea occurred to me that by the experimental ligation of the duct and the subsequent degeneration of a portion of the pancreas, that one might obtain the internal secretion free from the external secretion. I got up and wrote down the idea and spent most of the night thinking about it.[19]

Frederick Banting

Frederick Banting was born on a farm in Ontario, Canada, on November 14, 1891. The youngest of five children and an unremarkable student, Banting was six feet tall, shy, more serious and studious than most, but a good athlete. He had the manners of an unpolished country boy and in college spent much of his time with his girlfriend, Edith Roach.

Banting's medical studies were interrupted by World War I. He returned to Canada after the war, set up a medical practice, and planned to marry Edith once his practice made money. It never did. Banting took on extra work as a demonstrator at the medical school and, under pressure from Edith, searched for additional ways to earn a living. J.J.R. Macleod's offer of lab space gave Banting an excuse to leave his unsuccessful medical practice. Banting arrived in Toronto with little money and no promise of a salary.

Banting's insulin days were a roller coaster of emotions, from extreme highs when the work was going well to frustration, depression, and paranoia when there were problems. In addition, his relationship with Edith was rocky, he had little money to live on, and Macleod was unwilling to devote resources to the project.

With the discovery of insulin, Banting became a folk hero. From humble roots he had become the first Canadian to receive a Nobel Prize. Although sought after as a celebrity, Banting never truly lost his shyness and never became a good public speaker.

Having a history of fights with Collip and Macleod, Banting matured and mellowed over time. He took up painting and became close friends with fellow insulin researcher Collip. However, Banting's antagonism toward Macleod remained undiminished.

Later, Banting devoted his efforts to finding a cure for cancer, but he never got the scientific training nor had time outside the public spotlight to make much headway. He was supportive of the students who clustered around him and established the Banting and Best Department of Medical Research at the University of Toronto.

Banting's Idea

Banting believed the pancreatic digestive juices (external secretion) might destroy the pancreatic hormone (internal secretion). Indeed, this might be the reason no one had been able to extract the hormone from the pancreas. Banting wondered if surgically tying off the pancreatic ducts and blocking the external secretion might solve this problem. Stopping the flow of pancreatice digestive juices was known to cause the cells producing the external secretion to shrivel up and the pancreas to atrophy. Only the islets of Langerhans would be left. Banting believed that under these conditions the pancreatic hormone could be extracted without fear of damage from the external secretion.

The next day, Banting shared his idea with F.R. Miller, a professor and neurophysiologist at Western University. Miller advised Banting to consult with John James Rickard Macleod, head of the Department of Physiology at the University of Toronto, who was well known for his work with carbohydrate metabolism.

On November 8, 1920, Banting met with J.J.R. Macleod to discuss his idea. Macleod was doubtful. Macleod was well aware of the trouble other researchers had had trying to prepare a pancreatic extract that would reduce the symptoms of diabetes. He was also aware of Forschbach's theory that extracts of the pancreatic hormone caused severe reactions in humans. In addition, Macleod doubted that Banting, who was woefully ignorant of the research in this area, would succeed where others had failed. However, since little work had been done with atrophied pancreases, Macleod agreed to give Banting space in his laboratory for eight weeks, ten experimental dogs, and a medical student to assist him. Banting remembers Macleod saying, "it was worth trying. . . . Negative results would be of great physiological value."[20]

Beginning the Research

When Banting arrived at the University of Toronto mid-May 1921, he met Charles H. Best, a student who had been asked to assist him. Macleod apparently had warned Best that the "[the research] would likely all go up in smoke but it would be a good operative training and [as scientists] we must leave no sod unturned."[21] Best had just completed an honors degree in physiology and biochemistry at the University of Toronto. The previous year he had studied diabetes in turtles and was familiar with techniques for measuring the sugar content of both blood and urine. This knowledge would enable Best to measure the effects of any pancreatic extract produced.

Best and Banting immediately got to work. Following Macleod's suggestion, Banting created diabetes in several dogs by removing their pancreases. This allowed Banting to learn the surgical technique and gave Best practice obtaining blood and urine sugar levels. In addition, it gave both Banting and Best a chance to study the course of diabetes in dogs.

Next, Banting operated on several other dogs, surgically tying off their pancreatic ducts to prevent production of the digestive enzyme. Once the dogs' pancreases had degenerated, either the degenerated pancreas would be implanted in a diabetic dog, or an extract of the degenerated pancreas would be given to a diabetic dog in the hope it would reduce the symptoms of diabetes.

Unsanitary Conditions

Banting and Best had trouble from the start. Conditions in the operating room were awful. The small room in the physiology department had not been used for surgery for more than ten years. Despite intense cleaning, it was hard to keep the operating room sterile. Banting wrote:

> The place where we were operating was not fit to be called an operating room. Aseptic work had not been done in it for some years. The floor could not be scrubbed properly, or the water would go through on the laboratories below. The walls could not be washed for they were papered and then yellow washed. There were dirty windows above the unsterilizable wooden operating table. The operating linen consisted of towels with holes in them.[22]

As a result, a number of the dogs developed infections and died. By the end of the first week, four of their ten experimental dogs were dead. By the end of the second week only three of the experimental dogs remained. Banting and Best began purchasing additional dogs on the streets of Toronto from those willing to sell. As Best remembers, "There were occasions when we made a tour through various parts of the city and bargained with owners of animals. They were paid for by funds we took from our own pockets."[23]

Progress and Problems

By mid-June, one month into the project, Banting and Best had been able to remove a dog's pancreas and observe the increase in blood sugar and sugar in the urine expected in a diabetic dog. Several dogs had had their pancreatic ducts surgically tied, and Banting and

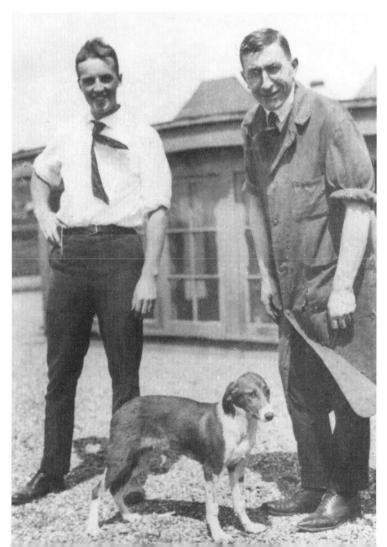

Best (left) and Banting pose with one of the dogs on which they experimented in search of an effective pancreatic extract.

Best were waiting for the dogs' pancreases to degenerate. In general, work was going according to the research plan. Macleod left for vacation to Scotland, leaving instructions for the next steps of the research, and Best went off for ten days of militia training, leaving Banting to continue the research alone.

Problems rapidly developed. Banting induced diabetes in another dog but could not get blood sugar or urine sugar measures that made sense. Another dog died on the operating table. By the time Best returned, Banting was frustrated and upset. Then came the extreme heat and humidity of the summer, which slowed the healing and recovery of the dogs. Finally, the duct-tying operations had to be repeated because the original operation worked properly in only two of the seven experimental dogs.

According to historian Michael Bliss, "The whole research program was not far from total failure. Banting and Best had experimented on nineteen dogs. Fourteen had died, no more than two of them according to the research plan. There were five duct-tied dogs left, and only two of them had gone according to plan."[24] It was mid-July 1921. The allotted eight weeks had passed.

Making Pancreatic Extract

Banting and Best continued despite their problems and disappointments. On July 30, 1921, they decided to put the theory about degenerated pancreases to the test. Instead of implanting the degenerated pancreas into a diabetic dog, they decided to go with the easier and quicker procedure of making an extract of the degenerated pancreas. Banting and Best described the procedure for making the extract as follows:

> The degenerated pancreas was swiftly removed and sliced into a chilled mortar containing Ringer's solution [artificial blood]. The mortar was placed in freezing mixture and the contents partially frozen. The half frozen gland was then completely macerated [ground up]. The solution was

filtered through paper and the filtrate [remaining liquid], having been raised to body temperature, was injected intravenously [into the diabetic dog's vein].[25]

An hour after injecting the extract into the first diabetic dog, the dog's blood sugar dropped by 40 percent. When the researchers injected the dog every hour, the dog's blood sugar remained much the same. When the researchers withheld the extract for two hours, the dog's blood sugar started to rise. At this point Banting and Best gave the dog sugar water through a stomach tube and the dog's blood sugar rose further. More extract given every hour did not reduce the blood sugar level, but no sugar appeared in the dog's urine and the increase in blood sugar was less than it would have

Pictured is the laboratory at the University of Toronto where Best and Banting engaged in their groundbreaking research.

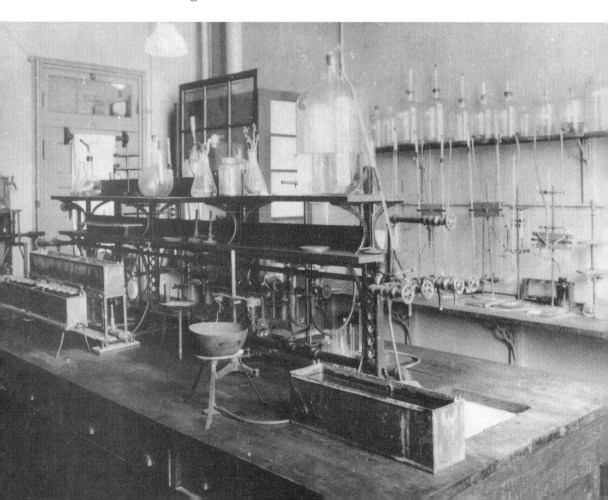

been without the extract. The results were unclear, but Best wrote Macleod, who was still in Scotland, that "the extract seemed to have a marked effect."[26]

Banting and Best tried the extract with another diabetic dog the next day. Again they saw the dog's blood sugar fall. A note in the lab book remarked that the dying dog was able to stand and walk after the first injection of extract. The dog's blood sugar fell even more after a second injection, but an hour later the dog was dead.

Banting and Best continued giving diabetic dogs extracts from degenerated pancreases. They observed

Charles Herbert Best

Charles H. Best was born on February 27, 1899, in West Pembroke, Maine. By the age of seven, Best would take care of the horses and harness a new team while his father, a country doctor, grabbed a bite to eat between visiting patients. Best was a lively, mischievous child but was also hardworking, modest, and generally well liked. Best had just completed an honors degree in physiology and biochemistry when he became Frederick Banting's assistant.

The study of diabetes held a special significance for Best after the death of his aunt in 1917. She had not only helped his father through medical school but also served as his father's nurse for a time, and her death from diabetes had a profound impact on him. However, Best could never have imagined where his work with Banting on diabetes would lead. Even before he had finished medical school, Best was famous as one of the discoverers of insulin. In October 1923 he was introduced to an auditorium overflowing with medical students at Harvard as the greatest medical student in the world and was credited for supplying the science needed to pursue Banting's idea. By his fifth year of medical school, Best was in charge of developing insulin for commercial use at the University of Toronto's Connaught Anti-Toxin Laboratories.

Best went on to graduate near the top of his class in 1925, and at the age of twenty-nine took J.J.R. Macleod's place as head of the Department of Physiology at the University of Toronto. There Best continued his work on insulin but also studied choline, an essential nutrient, and succeeded in isolating heparin, a compound that prevents blood from clotting.

In his later years, Best also directed the Banting and Best Department of Medical Research and was showered with honors. Although he did not receive the Nobel Prize, Best lived to see the authors of the official history of the Nobel Prizes conclude that a mistake had been made and Best should have shared the prize with Banting and Macleod. Charles Best retired in 1967.

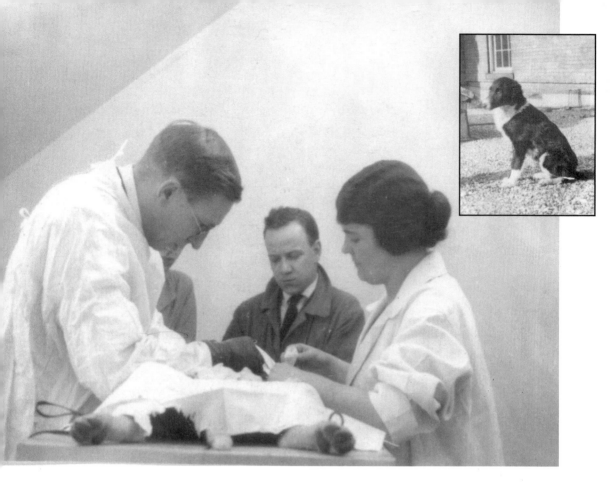

a marked decrease in the blood sugar of one dog injected with the pancreatic extract, but extracts of the spleen
and liver had no effect. Boiled extract also did not
reduce the dog's blood sugar level. It seemed the pancreatic extract was the only thing that worked.

Banting wrote Macleod, "The extract invariably causes a reduction in blood sugar, it improves the clinical
condition of the dog, it can be kept active for at least four
days."[27] Macleod wrote back, "You know, that if you can
prove *to the satisfaction of everyone* that such extracts really have the power to reduce blood sugar in pancreatic
diabetes, you will have achieved a very great deal."[28]

Not Enough Extract

In mid-August Banting and Best ran a control experiment. They used two diabetic dogs, giving the extract
to only one of them. The dog without the extract died;
the other dog made history, recovering to become a

Banting removes the pancreas of dog 33 (inset). Using a pancreatic extract, Banting and Best managed to keep the dog alive for seventy days.

In the fall of 1921 biochemist James B. Collip worked to purify Banting and Best's pancreatic extract for use on human diabetics.

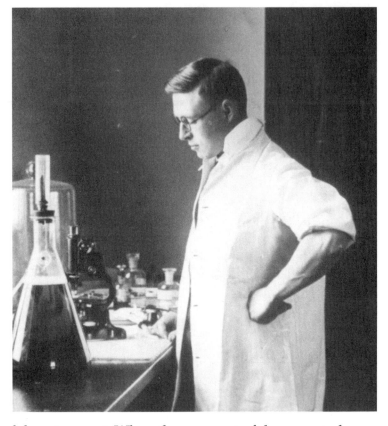

laboratory pet. When they ran out of degenerated pancreases, Banting and Best tried making extracts of whole pancreases. The whole pancreatic extracts worked even better than the degenerated pancreatic extracts, but Banting and Best were too exhausted from their efforts to notice.

Banting and Best continued to pursue extracts of degenerated pancreases, but they were out of dogs whose pancreatic ducts had been tied off. Needing more extract to keep their diabetic dogs alive, they developed a technique to exhaust the pancreas so it stopped producing the external secretion. They then made more extract from the exhausted pancreas.

Banting and Best were producing a pancreatic extract that kept diabetic dogs alive for days, but there were problems with their technique. First, the effects of the extract were not lasting. The blood sugar level stayed low only as long as the dog received more extract. Second, it took extracts from the pancreases of many healthy dogs to keep one diabetic dog alive. For example, it had taken the pancreases of five dogs to keep dog 92 alive for eight days. In short, the extract was impractical.

A New Source

In desperation Banting and Best turned to another source of pancreases. Banting had grown up on a farm and knew that cows were often bred to increase their weight prior to slaughter. He also knew that the pancreases of very young animals consist mostly of islet cells. If Banting could get the pancreases of fetal calves, he and Best would have a source of pancreas that was mostly islet cells.

Banting and Best's trip to the slaughterhouse was successful. Extract made from fetal calf pancreas worked to reduce blood sugar in diabetic dogs. Still, the supply of pancreas from fetal calves was limited. Following a suggestion made by Macleod, Banting and Best tried extracting the pancreatic enzyme from

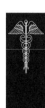

James Bertram Collip

Born in Ontario, Canada, in 1892, Bert Collip was the son of a florist of British descent. Shy and sensitive, Collip graduated college at the age of fifteen. He received his doctorate in biochemistry in 1916, and by 1920 he had been promoted to full professor in charge of the new department of biochemistry at the University of Alberta in Edmonton. Although he had a heavy teaching load at the University of Alberta, Collip's true love was research. He loved spending long hours in the laboratory, often at night, mixing this and that together to produce physiological reactions. He was on sabbatical at the University of Toronto when he agreed to refine the pancreatic extract produced by Best and Banting. Collip's extract was the first successful clinical use of insulin. Collip returned to the University of Alberta when his sabbatical ended and went on to become Canada's dominant figure in endocrinology, isolating one hormone after another. He ended his career as dean of medicine at the University of Western Ontario.

easily available cattle pancreas using techniques previously developed by Scott and Zuelzer. The process worked.

With a more accessible source of pancreas, Banting and Best managed to keep dog number 33, nicknamed Marjorie, alive without a pancreas for seventy days, sixty days longer than dog 33 could have survived on her own with diabetes. To prove that the extract had kept the dog alive, an independent pathologist performed an autopsy to look for any sign that dog 33's pancreas had not been completely removed. The pathologist found only a tiny fragment of pancreas that analysis showed contained no islet of Langerhans cells. The fragment could not have kept dog 33 alive; her longevity had to be due to the pancreatic extract. It looked like Banting and Best had found something that worked for diabetic dogs. Could it also work for humans?

Refining Insulin

In the fall of 1921 Macleod finally agreed to Banting's long-standing request that James Bertram Collip, a well-trained biochemist on sabbatical at the University of Toronto, join the team. Collip had an interest in internal secretions and more research experience than Banting and Best combined. Although Best was not happy about having a senior researcher take over his work of making the pancreatic extract, it helped with the workload, which was intensifying as interest grew in their results.

Collip was just what the team needed. He had a knack for what Collip himself called bathtub chemistry, and he was happy to mix, evaporate, distill, and tinker to find the best method for purifying a compound. Later, Collip's skill at extracting hormones would make him a legend in Canadian medical research.

Collip's task was to build on Best's work and create a purified extract that could be tried with human patients. In Collip's words, "The problem was to remove most of the protein and salts and all of the lipoid [fatty] material from the extracts without destroying the active principle."[29]

Collip was using rabbits to test his extract. As the extract became purer and thus stronger, some of the rabbits would have convulsive seizures and collapse into a coma. A graduate student witnessed Collip's reaction when the first rabbit had a seizure after receiving the extract. Apparently Collip's first thought was that there was something toxic in the extract. Then, remembered the graduate student, "[Collip] took a blood sample and set it aside, emptied solid glucose into water, shook it about, and injected it. The rabbit recovered shortly. Subsequent analysis of the blood indicated virtual absence of glucose. . . . It was the most thinking per square meter per minute that I have ever seen."[30]

Collip and the graduate student had witnessed what we now call insulin shock, the severe reaction that occurs when too much insulin causes blood sugar to fall to dangerously low levels. Using this knowledge, Collip went on to develop a method for testing the potency of pancreatic extracts using rabbits. He would adapt this method to test a purified extract for human use.

CHAPTER 4

Behind the Scenes

The pressure on the discoverers of the pancreatic hormone—soon to be named insulin—was intense. There was conflict among members of the research team. There were problems meeting the demand for the extract. The decision to award the Nobel Prize to J.R.R. Macleod and Frederick Banting, bypassing Charles H. Best and James Bertram Collip, only made matters worse. However, despite the struggles and obstacles, insulin would be produced commercially, saving the lives of thousands.

Sharing the Results

The first public presentation of Banting and Best's results took place November 14, 1921. The paper was given at a meeting of the University of Toronto's Physiology Journal Club, with Banting presenting and Best showing charts of their results. Macleod introduced the two men. Banting later complained, "Professor Macleod in his remarks gave everything that I was going to say and used the pronoun 'we' throughout. The following day, students were talking about the remarkable work of Professor Macleod."[31]

It was after this presentation that Macleod began assigning others in his lab to assist Banting and Best. Macleod also wrote to Dr. Elliott P. Joslin, one of the leading physicians treating diabetic patients, saying that the work looked promising but there were still some questions to be answered before the pancreatic extract could be considered for human use.

Best prepared a paper based on the November 14, 1921, presentation and submitted it to the *Journal of Laboratory and Clinical Medicine*, which published it on February 22, 1922. Word was starting to get out about Banting and Best's success.

Banting (below) kept detailed notes on his work. This page from his notebook reports a drop in dog 92's blood sugar after the dog received an injection of pancreatic extract.

December 30, 1921

On December 30, 1921, many of the important people working on diabetes attended Banting's presentation at the American Physiological Society at Yale University, including Joslin and Frederick Allen, another leading diabetologist in North America, and Israel Kleiner and Ernest Scott, both of whom had made significant contributions to the research on pancreatic extracts. Banting was nervous and spoke haltingly. In Banting's words, "When I was called upon to present our work I became almost paralyzed. I could not remember nor could I think. I had never spoken to an audience of this kind before—I was overawed. I did not present it well."[32]

In fact it was Macleod who came to the rescue. Realizing Banting had not convinced the audience that their research results proved that the long-sought pancreatic hormone existed, Macleod stepped in to answer questions. Joslin, writing years later, said, "Dr. Banting spoke haltingly, but we could gather that really something had happened and that the sugar in the blood of a dog had dropped. It was a little difficult to catch the whole story, but later this was emphasized and beautifully told by Dr. Macleod."[33]

Banting remembers his trip home from the meeting: "I did not sleep a wink on the train that night—I did not even go to my berth but sat up in the smoker condemning Macleod as an imposter and myself as a nincompoop. . . . It was foolish to spend weeks and months working night and day at experiments and then have them told beautifully by someone else who had the art as though they were his ideas and works."[34]

First Human Use

Fear that his work was being stolen out from under him may have spurred Banting to move forward with human testing. To be sure the extract was safe for humans, Banting injected first himself and then Best with the extract. Best remembered: "The next morning we had rather red arms, but there was no other effect. We did not follow our own blood sugars. However, we did test the material on one of our diabetic dogs and obtained a fine fall [drop in blood sugar] . . . thus we established the potency of this extract."[35]

On January 11, 1922, the extract Best had prepared was sent to Toronto General Hospital. It was given to Leonard Thompson, a fourteen-year-old boy with diabetes who weighed only sixty-four pounds and was close to death. Thompson was given two injections of what those present described as a thick brown muck. He developed abscesses at the injection sites and became even sicker, but tests showed his blood sugar level had dropped slightly. Although the extract lowered Thompson's blood sugar, the negative effects were too severe. Thompson's doctors stopped the treatment. The extract was not yet ready to be tested on humans.

Refining the Extract

Collip continued working to purify the extract. In the late evening of January 16, 1922, he finally found what he was looking for. He had discovered the conditions under which the hormone would not stay dissolved in the solution. The small, solid particles that formed were the most pure and concentrated version of the pancreatic extract to date. Collip wrote, "I experienced then and there all alone in the top story of the old Pathology Building perhaps the greatest thrill which has ever been given me to realize."[36]

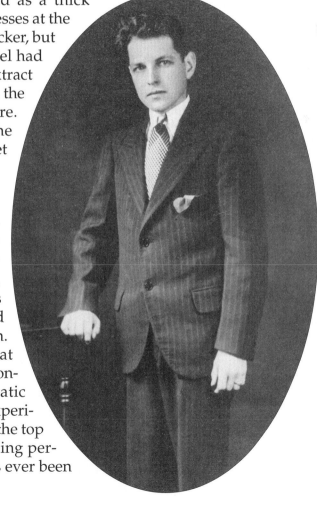

In January 1922 Leonard Thompson, a Canadian, became the first person to be treated for diabetes with insulin.

The Impact of Insulin

Dr. Elliot P. Joslin, in "Reminiscences of the Discovery of Insulin," wrote of his initial experiences using insulin to treat patients. Dr. Joslin was one of the leading diabetologists in the United States at the time insulin was discovered.

For a quarter of a century I had been treating, or rather fighting diabetes, when I heard a rumor of a surprising discovery by two young men in Toronto and went to New Haven in December 1921 to hear Banting speak about his experiment before the American Physiological Society. . . . A few months later Banting and Best . . . showed us their early cases, but the full impact of the discovery did not fully dawn upon me until I learned I was to receive insulin for trial with my own patients. I remember well staying awake all night the day before it was to arrive. The first unit I gave to Miss Madge, my severest patient, a nurse, on August 7, 1922. She had obeyed the rigid regime. During her five years of diabetes her weight had fallen from 157 to 72 pounds, but she remained sugar free. She was nearly bedridden and, I recall, had gone over [used] a flight of stairs in her home . . . but once in nine months. I watched her come back to life and go on in later years to care for her mother instead of her mother's taking care of her. After four weeks of insulin, she walked four miles, and in seven months she gained twenty pounds. She lived another twenty-five years.

Collip tested the potency of the new extract on rabbits. When the rabbits did not develop any abscesses, Collip was convinced he finally had a pancreatic extract that was ready for human use. He sent the refined extract over to the hospital, and on January 23, 1922, Leonard Thompson was given Collip's new extract, with much better results. Within twenty-four hours, Thompson's blood sugar level fell to normal. With the help of Collip's new extract, Thompson rapidly gained weight and strength. The original testing on Thompson had been rushed, but this second trial proved successful.

Conflict

It is unclear whether Collip was annoyed that Banting insisted Best prepare the first extract for clinical use insted of Collip. In any event, less than a week after Best's extract was given to Leonard Thompson, Collip entered the lab and, according to Best, "announced to me that he was leaving our group and that he intended to take out a patent in his own name on the improvement of our pancreatic extract. This seemed an extraordinary move to me, so I requested him to wait until Fred Banting appeared, and to make quite sure he did I closed the door and sat in a chair which I placed against it."[37]

Banting's memory of that evening provides further details:

> Collip had become less and less communicative and finally after about a week's absence he came into our little room about five-thirty one evening. He stepped inside the door and said, "Well, fellows, I've got it." I turned and said, "Fine, congratulations. How did you do it?" Collip replied, "I have decided not to tell you." His face was white as a sheet. He made as if to go. I grabbed him with one hand by the overcoat where it met in front and almost lifting him I sat him down hard on the chair. I do not remember all that was said but I remember telling him it was a good job he was so much smaller—otherwise I would "knock hell out of him." He told us that he talked it over with Macleod and that Macleod agreed with him that he should not tell us by what means he had purified the extract."[38]

Agreement

Back at the lab, Macleod finally realized something was wrong. He had noticed the tension between Banting and Best, on the one hand, and Collip, on the other. He had also heard reports that Banting was accusing him of stealing Banting's research. Something had to be done.

On January 25, 1922, an agreement was forged between Banting, Best, Collip, Macleod, and Connaught Anti-Toxin Laboratories, a branch of the University of Toronto devoted to producing vaccines and anti-toxins. The four researchers agreed that none of them would patent the extract. Instead they would cooperate with Connaught, which would pay for staff and equipment to develop the extract further. The open conflict simmered down, and the group focused on getting the extract ready for human use.

An Extract for Human Use

On February 11, 1922, Banting gave the extract to his friend and fellow physician Joe Gilchrist, a diabetic who was hanging on to life by following a starvation diet and exercising as much as he could manage. Banting and Best wanted to see if a person with diabetes could metabolize sugar better after receiving the extract. The immediate results were disappointing. However, several hours later, Joe Gilchrist started feeling better. It was easier to breathe, his head felt clear, and his energy increased. In Gilchrist's words, "It was as if I was walking on air. I hadn't felt like this in five years."[39] Similar tests at Toronto General Hospital confirmed the extract helped people with diabetes process sugars.

Disaster

Then disaster struck. To his and everyone else's surprise, Collip found he could not make the extract in large batches using the equipment set up by Connaught Anti-Toxin Laboratories. Worse, Collip began having trouble producing the refined extract in his laboratory as well. The amount of available extract for patients shrank and then dried up all together. Collip was working late into the night but could not produce extract that contained the active pancreatic hormone.

It was not unusual for scientists at that time to have trouble reproducing results when purifying unknown substances. Collip, working with crude and unreliable equipment, was hard put to control precisely each step of the extraction process. Changes in vacuum pressure, temperature, and distilling time can all affect biological substances. In addition, Collip had not kept careful notes on the process.

But the stakes were high. For two months no extract was available for clinical use. The most seriously ill patients at the hospital received whatever partially extracted material was available, but for one little girl it was not enough. She entered a coma in April 1922 and died. Meanwhile, the *Toronto Star* was publishing stories about the discovery at the university, and people were calling to beg for the extract.

Patenting

In April 1922 the Canadian team prepared a paper titled "The Effects Produced on Diabetes by Extracts of the Pancreas." This paper not only included the animal results but also discussed the effect of the extract on patients with diabetes. This time the extract was given a name, *insulin*, after the Latin word for island.

The paper was presented by Macleod at the American Association of Physicians on May 3, 1922. It was the closest yet to a formal announcement of the discovery of insulin. Although others also presented their research on pancreatic extracts in the same session, Dr. Frederick Allen said, "If, as seems to be the case, the Toronto workers have the internal secretion of the pancreas fairly free from the toxic material, they hold the unquestionable priority for one of the greatest achievements of modern medicine."[40]

Back in Toronto, Macleod was worried about the future of the team's work. The researchers had announced to the world the discovery of insulin but could not consistently produce the extract. What if other researchers managed to produce a good-quality extract before they did? What if someone else took out a patent and created a monopoly on production of the hormone? Both Macleod and Banting were determined that insulin be available to all who needed it.

In the end, they decided a patent was necessary. In Macleod's words, "I was at first opposed to the idea of taking out any patents whatsoever but was compelled to change my point of view when I saw that in no other way could we effectively control the proper manufacture and sale of insulin."[41] The patent was taken in the name of Banting, Best, and Collip for the University of Toronto. With the patent, the knowledge of how to make insulin would be available to all. The university would license manufacturers for a small royalty and that royalty would be used to fund research.

Production Resumes

Banting, Best, Collip, and Macleod all worked hard, although not without tension, throughout April and May to produce more extract. Each contributed ideas, and the four men functioned more effectively as a team than they had in some time. They narrowed the problem to a few steps in the production process and in

The Nobel Prize

Insulin was bringing dying patients back to life. The medical and scientific worlds were abuzz with the discovery, so it was no surprise that the discoverers of insulin were awarded a Nobel Prize. But, although Frederick Banting and Charles Best had discovered insulin, the 1923 Nobel Prize was given to Banting and J.J.R. Macleod.

There are several theories about how the prize was awarded. First, there was the issue of seniority. Macleod was an internationally known expert on carbohydrate metabolism, and the work on insulin had been done in his lab. If he had not participated directly in the initial work, he had nevertheless outlined preliminary experiments and worked to solidify the results once they showed promise. Best, on the other hand, was a young medical student and as such his contributions were assumed to be less substantial than those of the more senior members of the team.

Second, the Nobel Prize can be given to no more than three people for the same work, thus eliminating the possibility the prize could go to Banting, Best, James Collip, and Macleod. Finally, Nobel Prize recipients must be nominated. Banting received three nominations and Macleod two. Neither Best nor Collip nor any of the previous researchers—including E.L. Scott, Georg Zuelzer, and Nicolas Paulesco—had been nominated. Upon investigation, the Nobel Prize nominating committee concluded the idea and initial work were Banting's, but his success was due to Macleod's guidance. They decided to give both Banting and Macleod the 1923 Nobel Prize.

Furious that his coworker had been overlooked, Banting announced he would share his prize money with Best. Banting also praised Best in his acceptance speech. Macleod, wanting to acknowledge Collip's role, shared the prize money with him. Both Georg Zuelzer and Nicolas Paulesco protested the award and the lack of recognition for their work. The Nobel Prize committee never changes its awards, but years later the secretary of the 1923 Nobel Committee wrote that in hindsight, awarding the prize to Banting, Best, and Paulesco might have been the fair thing to do.

mid-May finally could make insulin once again. The new process used reagents that were expensive and extremely flammable. In hindsight Peter Moloney, a chemist on the Canadian team, remarked, "You can't imagine a more dangerous set-up."[42] The new process took several days to produce the extract, but it worked. Insulin was again available for clinical trials.

In early June 1922 Collip's sabbatical ended, and Best was left at Connaught Anti-Toxin Laboratories with responsibility for developing large-scale production of insulin. Banting's friend and colleague Joe Gilchrist became Best's human test subject, testing each batch of insulin on himself after it had been tried on the rabbits and before it was distributed for human use.

The Miracle of Insulin

Banting and Gilchrist also started treating patients at Toronto's Christie Street Military Hospital. As Paul de Kruif described in his 1932 book about great medical discoveries:

> Joe and his boys [the veterans at Christie Street Military Hospital] were a grand bunch of rabbits, all of them, those first days in May and June, 1922, when insulin was still crude and dangerous. From abscesses from its injection in their arms, their legs, their thighs got crosshatched with scars so you'd swear there was no place left to inject them. But they lived. They weren't starving any longer. Strength flowed back into these boys who'd become miserable objects of Government charity. . . . Jobs, the chance to earn their own livings, to be men again, this was all possible now. And they only laughed and never minded the terrible burning and pain of those early shots of insulin, while Best fixed and fixed at making it painless and safer.[43]

A nurse who worked with Dr. Allen's diabetic patients remembers the impact the news of insulin had on the hospital's patients: "The mere illusion of new hope cajoled patient after patient into new life. Diabetics who had not been out of bed for weeks

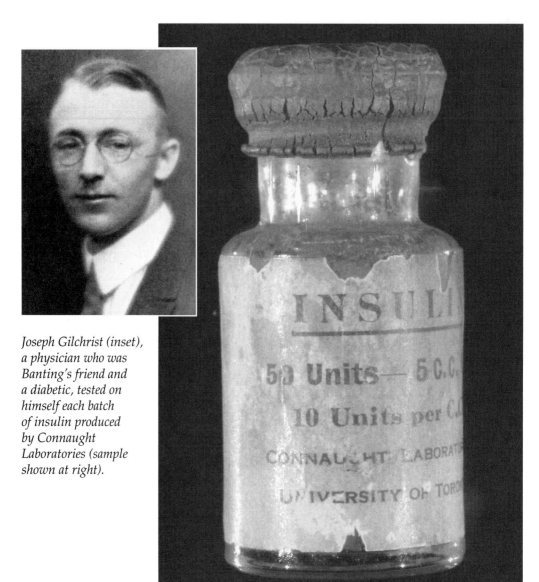

Joseph Gilchrist (inset), a physician who was Banting's friend and a diabetic, tested on himself each batch of insulin produced by Connaught Laboratories (sample shown at right).

began to trail weakly about, clinging to walls and furniture. Big stomachs, skin-and-bone necks, skull-like faces, feeble movements, all ages, both sexes—they looked like an old Flemish painter's depiction of a resurrection after famine."[44]

Insulin produced dramatic results. On May 21, 1922, James Havens Jr. became the first patient in the United

States to be treated with insulin. Havens was the son of the vice president of Eastman Kodak and had been diagnosed with diabetes when he was fifteen. He had done fairly well on Dr. Allen's undernutrition diet for seven years before he rapidly became worse. When news of the discovery of insulin arrived, Havens lay like a living skeleton in bed. He was barely able to lift his head and suffered from weakness, pain, hunger, and despair. Two weeks after receiving the correct dose of insulin, Havens was able to get out of bed and walk around.

In May 1922 James Havens Jr. became the first person in the United States to receive insulin.

Producing Insulin on a Larger Scale

As news of the success of insulin spread, thousands of patients and their families demanded treatment. Heartbreaking letters arrived begging for insulin. It was obvious more insulin was necessary to treat people with diabetes than Best and the others at Connaught Anti-Toxin Laboratories could produce. An experienced pharmaceutical house was needed to handle large-scale production.

On May 30, 1922, the Board of Governors of the University of Toronto entered into an agreement with the U.S. pharmaceutical company Eli Lilly and Company. For one year, Eli Lilly and its chemists would work alongside the Toronto team and share efforts to produce insulin on a large scale. To meet the clinicians' demands

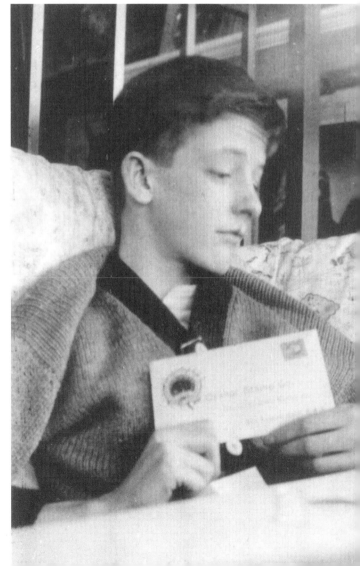

Letters of Entreaty and Thanks

Once the news about insulin spread, the Toronto team received many letters such as this one from the chief pediatrician at Johns Hopkins in Baltimore, Maryland, quoted in *The Discovery of Insulin* by Michael Bliss:

> I have some really heart-breaking cases under my care at the present time, two of them lone children of different families whose carbohydrate tolerance is gradually going down. They know of your work and are pestering me to get some of the material if I can. I do not wish to pester you, but only to let you know how anxious I am to use some of the insulin if I can get it.

Patients wrote, too. In Best's book, *Margaret and Charley*, eight-year-old Frederick Gerrier wrote a letter from the hospital: "Dear Doctors, I want to thank you for making serum [insulin]. It has helped me along well. I am getting lots more to eat and am feeling better." Patrick W. Coffey, a father of two little boys, wrote to say that insulin's control of his diabetes not only made him feel better, but had improved the life of his whole family. Richard Whitner stated: "I have almost starved to death, and now to be able to have enough food to satisfy makes me so thankful and grateful to you." Perhaps fourteen-year-old Elizabeth Hughes's letters home to her mother best sum up the feelings of those first days of insulin. She wrote: "To think that I'll be leading a normal, healthy existence is beyond all comprehension. Oh, it is simply too wonderful for words this stuff [insulin]."

they agreed that a select group of physicians and institutions would be given the extract for testing purposes as soon as it became available. At the end of the year, Eli Lilly would be given the same rights as other manufacturers to produce insulin; Eli Lilly's rights would be limited to North, Central, and South America.

In the meantime, W.D. Sansum of the Potter Metabolic Clinic in Santa Barbara, California, had begun producing insulin for his patients using the methods published by the Canadian team. Other researchers and clinicians flocked to Toronto to learn how to produce insulin, and the Canadian team shared their knowledge. Still, the supply of insulin was limited.

In 1922 the insulin produced by the Toronto group still contained protein impurities that caused pain and abscesses at the injection site. Eli Lilly's extracts were purer, but the potency of the insulin could vary up to

25 percent from batch to batch. Just as Eli Lilly was gearing up to make larger quantities of insulin, the U.S. government forced a change in the type of alcohol the company was allowed to use. Then, in early August, several batches were produced that had no active insulin. In response, the company set aside its efforts to manufacture large quantities and went back to producing enough insulin for the patients currently using it.

It was not until late 1922 that George Walden, chief chemist at Eli Lilly, realized the acidity of the extracting solution was a key factor in the production process. Looking more closely at the problem, Walden realized the active principle (the hormone named insulin) fell out of solution and formed a solid substance when the solution was within a certain range of acidity. With less active principle in the solution, the extract had little potency. Recognizing the solid substance contained a purer form of the hormone, Walden set up an extraction process that used the solid substance and produced, in Walden's words, "a product having a stability many times as great and a purity ranging from ten to one hundred times as great as the best product hitherto obtainable."[45] Using Walden's new method, Eli Lilly solved its production problem. By February 1923 Eli Lilly was able to produce huge reserves of insulin. The treatment of diabetes had entered a new era.

CHAPTER 5

Insulin and Technology Today

People with type 1 diabetes need insulin to live. Many people with type 2 diabetes use insulin to maintain normal blood sugar levels. In the early days, insulin injections were painful and the dosage difficult to calculate. Since people with diabetes can suffer fatal complications if their blood sugar is too high (hyperglycemia) or falls too low (hypoglycemia), there has been a tremendous push to make using insulin easier. Today various forms of insulin and new technologies help people with diabetes maintain their blood sugar levels within a normal range.

A New Era

With the availability of insulin, treatment of diabetes entered a new era. No longer was diabetes a death sentence or at best a life of starvation. The use of insulin enabled people with diabetes to lead fairly normal lives. In fact, Elizabeth Evans Hughes, among the first to receive insulin, did not tell her fiancé she had diabetes until they were about to be married.

Life expectancy for a ten-year-old child diagnosed with diabetes rose from 1.3 years in 1897 to 45 years in 1945. Although people with diabetes needed daily injections of insulin and had to watch their diets, insulin seemed a miraculous cure. Physician Frank N. Allan noted the change in Leonard Thompson, the first person to receive Best and Banting's extract: "Three years later, when I was an intern in the Toronto General Hospital, I saw Leonard Thompson when he came in regularly to secure his supply of insulin. He was now a sturdy young man, who showed little resemblance to the emaciated, dying boy who had been the subject of the most crucial clinical experiment in the field of diabetes."[46]

Despite the dramatic recovery insulin provided people with diabetes, insulin was not easy to use. The potency and purity of insulin batches varied, making estimating the correct dosage difficult. Doctors kept candy, orange juice, or injectable glucagon (a hormone that releases sugar stored in the liver) on hand in case

Hypoglycemia, Insulin Shock, and Hyperglycemia

Hypoglycemia occurs when a person's blood sugar level drops too low. Symptoms can include sweating; confusion; dizziness or light-headedness; hunger; feeling shaky, nervous, or anxious; having a headache; tingling around the lips; pale skin; nausea; slurred speech; rapid heart rate; clumsy or jerky movements; or seizures. If left untreated, hypoglycemia may lead to unconsciousness and death. The symptoms can be treated with juice, candy, or glucose tabs. If unconscious, the victim can be given an injection of glucagon, which will cause the liver to release glucose. If hypoglycemia occurs because too much insulin has been taken or has built up in the body, it is often called insulin shock.

On the other hand, high blood sugar, or hyperglycemia, occurs when there is too much glucose in the bloodstream. The immediate effects of high blood sugar include thirst, frequent urination, blurred vision, fatigue, and weight loss. If high blood sugar continues without treatment, it can lead to diabetic coma and death. Over time, high blood sugar levels can damage nerves, producing numbness, tingling, burning, prickling, or aching sensations. Loss of nerve function can also disrupt bodily functions such as digestion. Another effect of hyperglycemia, the narrowing of large blood vessels, can cause heart attacks and strokes. Narrowed blood vessels also reduce blood circulation, making it harder for cuts and sores to heal and increasing the chance for serious infections and amputation of a limb. Damage to the small blood vessels from hyperglycemia can cause blurred vision, blindness, and kidney disease.

a strong batch of insulin produced hypoglycemia or insulin shock after injection.

In addition, the first patients were injected with five to ten milliliters (one to two teaspoons) of insulin at a time. Typically, injections were given under the skin of the buttocks, thighs, or upper arms. Pain and abscesses at the injection site were common.

Doctors tried having patients swallow insulin instead, but the digestive juices of the stomach destroyed the active ingredient. Rectal administration also proved ineffective. Some doctors even withheld insulin for a time, hoping the patient's pancreas would work again after the rest provided by the initial treatment. All these approaches were to no avail. Only regular injections of insulin would reduce the blood sugar of patients with diabetes. Since people with diabetes would have to endure insulin injections several times a day for the rest of their lives, it was important to improve the purity of the insulin and reduce the volume of the injections.

Changes in Insulin

By February 1923 Eli Lilly was producing a purer form of insulin than the original version. The increased purity caused less pain and fewer abscesses at the injection site. Then, in 1926, J.J. Abel crystallized insulin, enabling an even purer form of the hormone to be made. Both versions of insulin acted quickly to lower blood sugar, but their effects lasted only four to six hours. People with diabetes needed multiple injections of insulin each day.

In the mid-1930s, long-acting protamine zinc insulin was developed. Now people with diabetes could get by with one injection a day. Given the discomfort and time it took to prepare and give an injection, taking only one injection appealed to many, but the long-lasting insulins still had problems.

With regular insulin, symptoms of hypoglycemia appear soon after injection of an insulin dose that is too large or too strong. Longer-lasting insulins act so slowly that the lowest blood sugar level and highest risk of seizures and death from hypoglycemia occur hours after injection. This makes timely reactions to insulin shock problematic. For example, hypoglycemia that occurs at night when the person is sleeping might induce seizures or a coma without anyone's notice. Daytime onset of hypoglycemia symptoms, such as slurred speech and clumsy, jerky movements, could be embarrassing if interpreted as drunkenness or dangerous if the person is driving.

Another long-lasting insulin, neural protamine Hagedorn (NPH), was introduced in the 1940s, followed by the lente series of insulin in the 1950s. The lente insulins last from twenty to thirty hours, thanks to the addition of a substance that slows down the body's absorption of insulin. In the 1960s and 1970s advances in chromatography allowed the production of purified insulin, including a highly purified form of insulin developed by the Danish called monocomponent insulin.

Beef, Pork, and Human Insulin

For many years all insulin was extracted from the pancreases of animals, mainly cattle in the United States and the United Kingdom and pigs in Denmark. Impurities in the insulin extracts were due to the presence of other compounds in the pancreases. In addition, although beef, pork, and human insulins differ from each other by only one to three amino acids, the sulfur connections between the two amino acid chains that compose insulin are in slightly different places. For some people, these minor differences can cause allergic reactions; other people develop resistance over time to beef or pork insulin.

With the development of DNA technology, it became possible to synthesize an insulin with the same amino acid sequence as human insulin. The first biosynthetic human insulin came out in 1983. In July 1996 the Food and Drug Administration approved the first recombinant DNA human insulin analogue, Humalog.

A diabetic injects a syringe full of insulin into his side. Today, synthesized human insulin is the most common type of insulin in use.

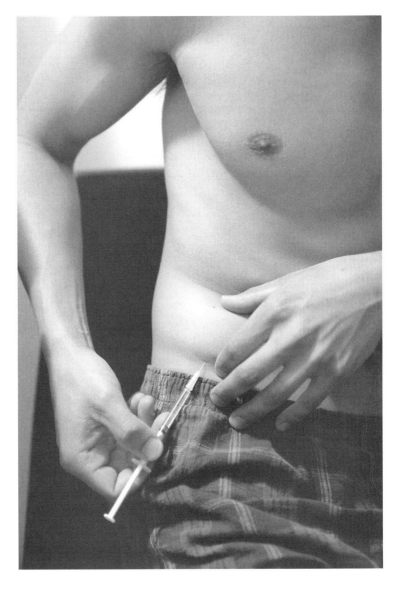

Today synthesized human insulin is practically the only insulin used. It does away with the need for massive quantities of animal pancreas and eliminates the potential for allergic reactions.

Not a Cure

Even with tremendous improvements in its quality, insulin is not a cure for diabetes. As historian Michael

Bliss notes, "It was gradually realized that insulin had not solved the problem of diabetes. Diabetics who got the insulin they needed and then balanced their diets and their insulin as carefully as possible were still not physiologically normal. Artificially supplied insulin could not perfectly compensate for the missing pancreatic function."[47]

A functioning pancreas continually responds to changes in blood sugar throughout the day, producing more insulin to digest food or to supply glucose to working muscles. It is impossible to mimic these continual internal adjustments with periodic injections of insulin. The inability to fine-tune blood sugar levels means that, over time, periods of high blood sugar take their toll. David Bjerklie, writing for *Time* magazine, noted, "Even with insulin . . . the complications of Type 1 [diabetes] can take a terrible toll. By age fifty-five, for example, 35% of victims have died of a heart attack. Kidney failure is also common, and after 15 years of the disease, 80% of Type 1 diabetics have sustained significant eye damage."[48]

Complications of Diabetes

With the help of insulin, more people with diabetes are living longer, but they are also experiencing complications of the disease, including blindness, nerve damage, heart disease, loss of circulation to the limbs, kidney failure, and increased risk of infections. Today diabetes is the leading cause of blindness among adults aged twenty to seventy-four. Diabetes is also responsible for 40 percent of patients with kidney failure, and 60 to 65 percent of people with diabetes have high blood pressure. Children who develop diabetes are still at two to three times the risk of dying prematurely.

According to Dr. David G. Orloff, director of the Food and Drug Administration's Division of Metabolic and Endocrine Drugs, "Daily monitoring and careful control of blood sugar levels are the most important steps people with diabetes can take. . . . Maintaining normal levels is difficult but good glycemic [blood sugar level]

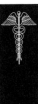

Testing Sugar Levels

Prior to the 1950s, sugar levels were checked with urine tests. In 1911 Stanley Benedict developed a simple color-coded way to test a diabetic's urine for sugar. Eight to ten drops of fresh urine were added to a test tube containing a teaspoon of Benedict's solution. The mixture was boiled for three minutes and then allowed to cool. The color of the cooled solution showed roughly how much sugar was present in the urine. If the solution was blue, there was no sugar in the urine. Green meant there was a trace of sugar. Yellow, orange, and red signified increasing amounts of sugar, with red indicating a dangerous level of sugar in the urine. People with diabetes had to repeat this test several times a day to determine how much insulin they needed to take. The result of each urine test was recorded in a log book so that the patient's doctor could see the urine sugar levels over time. The process was both time-consuming and nerve-racking.

By the mid-1950s simpler methods for testing urine sugar were being developed. Helen Murray Free first developed dry reagents that could test urine sugar levels and then went on to develop a convenient test for urine sugar. A test strip dipped into a sample of urine would quickly change color, giving an almost immediate measurement of urine sugar.

control is key to preventing long-term complications."[49] As one person with diabetes summed it up, "No news is not good news as a diabetic. The more we know about our condition, the better our condition."[50]

Monitoring Blood Sugar Levels

In recent years monitoring blood sugar has become easier. The urine tests of the past and the blood tests at the doctor's office have given way to blood glucose meters for home use. No longer do people with diabetes need to add eight to ten drops of fresh urine to a teaspoon of Benedict's solution (a commercial reagent) in a test tube, heat the mixture to a boil for three minutes, let it cool, and hope the color will show there is little or no sugar in the urine. Today people with diabetes need only prick their finger, smear the drop of blood onto a strip of special paper, and insert the paper into a machine called a blood glucose monitor that calculates the person's blood sugar level. Results from the blood glucose monitor come back quickly and accurately display the blood sugar levels.

Each year blood glucose meters become more sophisticated. Over one hundred new devices have been approved for sale in the past several years. Small and easily portable blood glucose meters make it easy to check blood sugar levels at school, work, or on the road. There are colorful models for children that give quick results, and large screens or talking models for people with vision problems. Some blood glucose meters can record the test results and track results over time, eliminating the need to maintain a hand-written log of each result.

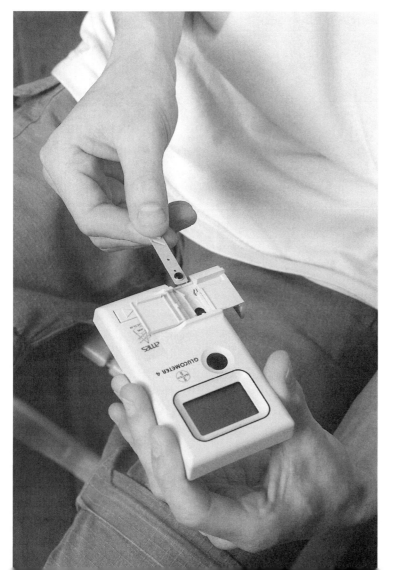

People with diabetes use a blood glucose monitor like this one to test their blood sugar levels. Over the years, monitoring techniques have dramatically improved.

Small, razor-sharp needles called lancets are used to prick a finger and obtain the drop of blood needed to test blood sugar. Today lancets come in many varieties. Spring-loaded lancets quickly prick the skin and are less painful. Some lancets can be set at specific prick depths for different thicknesses of skin. Portable battery-operated lasers can draw blood without using a lancet, and an arm patch is being developed that can draw glucose from under the skin to measure blood sugar.

In 2000 an all-in-one lancet and monitor came on the market; other models rapidly followed. These devices make checking blood sugar a one-step process and even eliminate the need for a finger prick. One semi-automated device includes a blood glucose meter that is placed on the upper arm, forearm, or thigh. It uses light suction to hold the skin in place while an integrated device pricks the skin, transfers the small amount of blood to a biosensor strip, and calculates the blood sugar level in less than a minute. Because these devices require less blood and take blood from an arm or thigh, the prick to get blood is typically less painful. The cost of the all-in-one lancet and monitor is within the price range for more traditional blood glucose monitors, although the cost of the biosensor strips may vary.

Continuous Monitoring

Wristwatch monitors are now available to help people with diabetes track their blood sugar throughout the day. These blood glucose meters detect blood sugar levels through the skin. A low-level electrical current draws fluid beneath the skin to a sensor pad on the back of the watch. Every ten to twenty minutes a blood sugar reading is taken, and an alarm sounds if the blood sugar level is too high or too low. Finger pricks are still necessary twice a day to calibrate the device, but with continuous monitoring it is easier to adjust meals, snacks, exercise, and insulin injections to maintain blood sugar within a normal range.

Still other devices are being developed, including a continuous glucose monitor designed for implantation under the skin of the lower chest or abdomen. The implant would measure blood glucose levels and transmit the information to a pagerlike device worn outside the body. Still another product under development is a near-infrared light beam that can shine through an earlobe, fingertip, or other body tissue packed with blood vessels and determine blood sugar levels from the concentration of sugar in the tissue.

New technology has also made it easier for doctors to help their patients. In 1999 the Continuous Glucose Monitoring System was approved for use. A small,

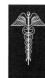

Blood Sugar Levels

Normal blood sugar falls within the range of 60 to 110 milligrams per deciliter (mg/dl). After a person eats, the blood sugar level will rise but will rarely reach beyond 180 mg/dl. How much blood sugar levels rise after eating depends upon the type of food consumed and the individual's own metabolic response.

People who are prediabetic have trouble bringing their blood sugar level down to the normal range after eating a meal that contains carbohydrates. The criteria for being prediabetic is having blood sugar levels between 110 and 126 mg/dl after fasting or between 140 to 200 mg/dl after taking the oral glucose tolerance test.

Diabetes is diagnosed when two blood sugar tests done on separate days after a twelve-hour fast show blood sugar levels equal to or greater than 126 mg/dl. In people with symptoms of diabetes, two nonfasting blood levels greater than or equal to 200 mg/dl confirms the presence of diabetes.

Left untreated, very high blood sugar levels of 360 mg/dl can be life-threatening. Having blood sugar readings at this level means that the body cannot use glucose for food; instead, it breaks down fat for fuel-releasing ketones. Ketones can disturb the body's acid/base balance, leading to a state called ketoacidosis that requires immediate medical attention.

At one time, people with diabetes were told to keep their blood sugar levels between 40 and 180 mg/dl, but this was not good enough to prevent complications of diabetes. Ideal levels were reset at 120–140 mg/dl, but the ten-year Diabetes Control and Complications Trial proved that maintaining near-normal blood sugar levels could reduce the risk of complications of diabetes by as much as 75 percent, so the ideal level was revised yet again. Currently people with diabetes strive to maintain their blood sugar levels at 70 to 90 mg/dl.

disposable glucose-sensing device is inserted beneath the skin and attached to a beeper-sized recording device. The sensor takes glucose levels every five minutes for up to three days. At the end of the allotted time, the data is downloaded by the doctor and combined with data from at least three finger prick tests per day and the individual's log of insulin doses, meals, and activities. This creates an almost minute-to-minute picture of how the person's blood sugar level varies thoughout the day. The doctor can then identify any problems and fine-tune the person's medication and diet so that the blood sugar level remains in the normal range around the clock.

Responding to Blood Sugar Levels

Along with new technology for measuring blood sugar, new developments have made responding to changes in blood sugar levels easier. For example, over twenty types of insulin are now available. The different insulins vary by how quickly they start to work, how long they take to become effective, and how long they continue to reduce blood sugar. Someone with diabetes can take an insulin that acts very quickly for a short period of time or an insulin that takes a while to act but lasts a long time. The choice depends on the individual's lifestyle and blood sugar patterns.

People with diabetes can also mix types of insulin so they will have a peak of insulin around the time they eat or plan heavy exercise and a lower level of insulin at other times of the day. Premixed versions of insulin eliminate the need to individually measure each type of insulin. These premixed versions are usually injected before breakfast and before the evening meal to accommodate the body's need for additional insulin at mealtime.

Methods for Taking Insulin

There have also been changes in the way people can take insulin. For decades people with diabetes have used a syringe with a needle to inject themselves. Today's small syringes with very thin needles make injections nearly painless. However, other alternatives are now available. Insulin pen injectors are syringes that look like a cartridge pen, but the cartridge is filled with insulin instead of ink. The dose is set with a dial, the needle inserted under the skin, and the click of a button at the end of the pen delivers the insulin. Not only does the pen offer a discreet way to inject insulin, but it is a handy way to carry insulin for routine injections or emergency backup. Prefilled cartridges can make the process even easier. Researchers are experimenting with a number of other delivery systems,

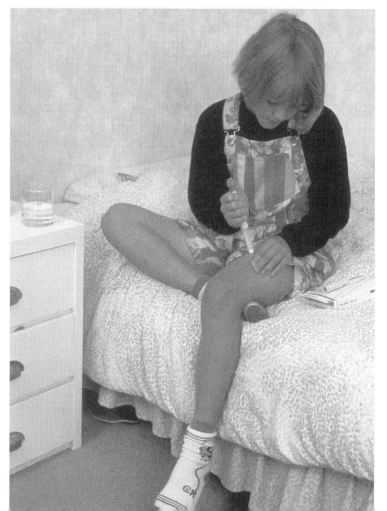

A diabetic girl injects insulin into her leg using a pen injector. This injection method is discrete, convenient, and virtually painless.

Pro golfer Michelle McCann wears an insulin pump (below) on her belt during a tournament. The pump delivers a steady insulin flow to her body.

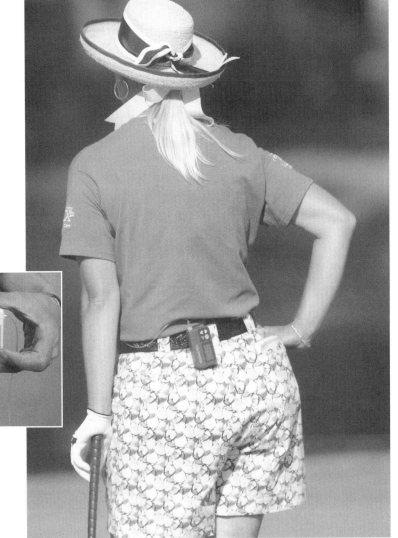

including nasal and mouth sprays, inhalers, and patches—in short, anything that could easily and accurately deliver insulin and do away with the need to take an injection.

Insulin jet injectors and infusers are alternatives to daily injections with a needle. Insulin jet injectors send a fine spray of insulin through the skin using highly pressurized air. Insulin infusers are flexible hollow tubes, or catheters, that a person inserts under the skin of their abdomen or hip. Daily doses of insulin are then injected into the infuser catheter instead of through the skin. After several days, the infuser is removed, and a new catheter is inserted in a different spot.

Insulin Pumps

Insulin pumps are another option. The pumps continuously deliver short-acting insulin, maintaining a baseline level of insulin that more closely mimics the role of a healthy pancreas. Worn outside the body like a pager or cell phone, the pump has a reservoir filled with insulin and a small flexible tube that connects to a catheter inserted under the skin of the abdomen. The pump pushes insulin through the catheter into the body following a program set by the doctor or the wearer.

Typically the pump is set to deliver low levels of insulin throughout the day. The wearer sets the pump to deliver additional insulin at mealtime based on the carbohydrate content of the meal. Additional insulin can be delivered when exercising or as needed based on daily blood sugar checks. Every few days, more insulin is added to the reservoir and the catheter moved to a different location. Insulin pumps have several advantages over taking multiple daily injections: They improve control over blood sugar levels and offer the wearer freedom from timing meals and exercise to correspond with peak levels of injected insulin. Indeed, many people with diabetes can achieve normal or near-normal blood sugar levels by using an insulin pump.

However, insulin pumps are not for everyone. To use an insulin pump a person must monitor blood sugar regularly and work closely with a doctor to program the device. There is a risk of infection at the catheter site, and it may be difficult to wear the insulin pump when swimming or playing contact sports. To address these concerns, researchers are experimenting with insulin pumps that can be implanted under the skin of the abdomen and remotely controlled.

The effort to develop better and easier ways to measure and control blood sugar continues. The ten-year Diabetes Control and Complications Trial (DCCT) sponsored by the National Institute of Diabetes and Digestive and Kidney Diseases showed that maintaining near-normal blood sugar levels could reduce the risk of complications by as much as 75 percent. Maintaining normal blood sugar, however, is not always easy. The amount of insulin needed varies with diet, especially the amount of carbohydrates eaten. Exercise and illness also affect blood sugar levels, and infections can send blood sugar levels soaring. Researchers continue to respond, creating new and better technology to help people with diabetes track and respond to changes in their blood sugar throughout the day.

CHAPTER 6

Future Hopes for a Cure

The miracle of insulin keeps people with diabetes alive and living normal lives, but it is not a cure. People with diabetes continue to suffer from complications of the disease. Despite increasing knowledge about diabetes and how insulin works, the number of people with diabetes in the United States increases each year. The growing epidemic is putting pressure on researchers to find a cure for diabetes and regenerate a person's ability to produce insulin and regulate blood sugar.

Enhancing the Body's Ability to Produce Insulin

Not all people with diabetes depend on daily injections of insulin to stay alive. More than 90 percent of the people with diabetes in the United States have type 2 diabetes. Rather than taking insulin injections, these people mostly take oral medications to either boost the pancreas's production of insulin or help reduce the impact of the body's resistance to insulin.

Since World War II, oral medications called sulfonylureas have been used to stimulate the beta cells of the pancreas to produce more insulin. To address problems with hypoglycemia, several new versions of these drugs have been developed: Glipizide (Glucotrol) and glyburide (DiaBeta, Glynase, Micronase) are the most commonly used sulfonylureas today. These new medications do not last as long in the body and therefore reduce the risk that the drug will build up in the body, cause too much insulin to be produced, and send the user into insulin shock.

Also being developed is a class of drugs chemically different from the sulfonylureas. These drugs, called meglitinides, cause a rapid but short-lasting release of insulin by the pancreas. They are taken with meals to provide the extra insulin needed to process food. The quick action of these drugs and their rapid loss of effect mimic the mealtime production of insulin by a functioning pancreas. Since the effects of these drugs do not last, there is also less risk of hypoglycemia. One such drug, repaglinide (Prandin), has already been approved, and others are expected to be approved shortly.

Enhancing the Body's Ability to Respond to Insulin

Still other drugs address the problem of the body's resistance to insulin. The class of drugs called biguanides fit this mold. Metformin (Glucophage), the

Glycosylated Hemoglobin, or Hemoglobin A^{1C}

Hemoglobin is the protein within the blood that carries oxygen to cells throughout the body. When blood sugar attaches to the surface of the hemoglobin, it creates a slightly different form of hemoglobin called glycosylated hemoglobin, or hemoglobin A^{1C}. The amount of sugar that attaches to a person's hemoglobin depends upon how much sugar there is in the blood. Since the attachment occurs slowly, the amount attached will not change if there is a sharp rise or fall in blood sugar that does not last for an extended period of time. However, high blood sugar levels that last for several weeks will increase the amount of attached sugar.

There is now a test that can calculate the ratio of glycosylated hemoglobin to regular hemoglobin. This ratio provides information on the average blood sugar level over a period of time and gives a clearer measure of how well controlled the blood sugar level is on average, despite any peaks or valleys that may have occurred.

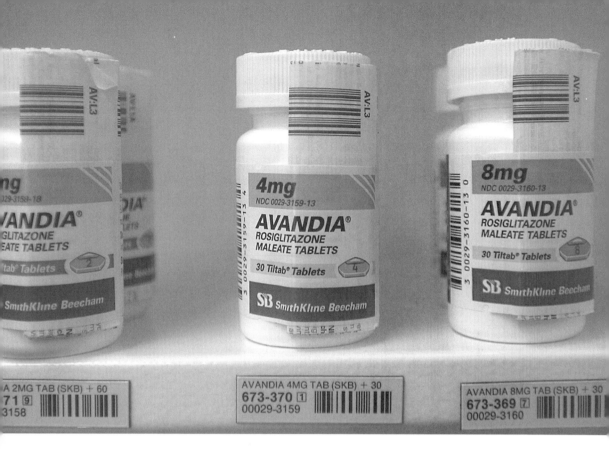

only biguanide available in the United States, seems to work by reducing the amount of sugar the liver releases between meals. It also appears to help glucose enter the cells of the liver and muscles—in other words, to help the insulin produced by the pancreas work more effectively.

Another class of drugs, the alpha-glucosidase inhibitors, slow digestion of carbohydrates. By delaying the breakdown of carbohydrates into sugar, the alpha-glucosidase inhibitors slow the normal rise of blood sugar after a meal. They also prevent sugar products from being absorbed by the intestine. This both reduces the overall amount of sugar and increases the time over which the sugar enters the bloodstream. Because alpha-glucosidase inhibitors spread out the peak in blood sugar normally seen after a meal, the available insulin has more time to do its job. Alpha-glucosidase inhibitors are typically taken with meals and are used for people with type 2 diabetes, whose

Rosiglitazone is one of the medications that help people with type 2 diabetes more effectively use the insulin their bodies produce.

blood sugar levels are highest after meals. Acarbose (Precose) and miglitol (Glyset) are the drugs currently available in this class.

The newest family of drugs designed to help type 2 diabetics are the thiazolidinediones. These include pioglitazone hydrochloride (Actos) and rosiglitazone (Avandia). These drugs make the tissues more sensitive to insulin, enabling the body to better use the insulin it produces. They also increase the liver's ability to store glucose. They work by enhancing the natural action of insulin in the body to help people with type 2 diabetes maintain a normal blood sugar level.

Limitations of Medication

Oral medications for people with type 2 diabetes work to enhance the body's ability to make and use insulin. They may prevent the need to inject insulin, but they are not cures for diabetes. Not only that, they can have negative effects. For example, some thiazolidinediones have caused liver damage or stimulated the growth of other organs, including the heart. A person can develop a tolerance to the medication so that it loses its effectiveness over time, and there is the constant risk of hypoglycemia. There is also a tendency to believe taking medication will control the disease. Dr. Richard S. Beaser and Joan V.C. Hill, authors of *The Joslin Guide to Diabetes*, note: "Sometimes the failure of diabetes pills is due not to the medications themselves, but because of 'user error.' People often make the mistake of abandoning their meal plan or exercise program, believing the tablets alone will handle their diabetes. But as effective as these pills may be, they can't take care of your diabetes themselves."[51] Nor can the oral medications regenerate the ability to control blood sugar internally.

Finding a Cure

With new surgical techniques and the rise of genetic engineering, hopes for developing a cure grow. Organ transplant is one potential option. Theoretically, a healthy pancreas implanted in a person with diabetes could take over the production and regulation of insulin, responding as needed to changes in blood sugar.

In 1966 the first patient received a transplanted pancreas. More surgeries followed, but the survival rate was discouragingly low and not many transplants were attempted. By 1978, however, new surgical techniques and medications improved the survival rate. Over twenty thousand patients worldwide have received transplanted pancreases; about fourteen hundred patients in the United States receive a pancreatic transplant each year.

Most pancreatic transplants are done in conjunction with, or following, a kidney transplant. Kidney failure is a common complication of diabetes, and receiving a pancreas in conjunction with a kidney may actually improve chances the kidney will survive. In addition, for patients whose pancreatic transplant is successful, the new pancreas produces insulin and regulates blood sugar, curing the patient's diabetes.

A patient's body, however, may reject the new pancreas as something foreign to the body. Anti-rejection drugs are available, but these drugs must be taken for life and have more negative effects than continual injections of insulin do. Thus, if insulin is working, there is little justification for taking the risks associated with surgery and pancreatic transplants. Christopher D. Saudek, president of the American Diabetes Association, notes, "[Pancreatic transplant] surgery is so major and the need for continuous immune suppression is more dangerous than taking insulin."[52]

To date, pancreatic transplants for people with diabetes have been performed only on those receiving kidney transplants or on those who are otherwise healthy but whose diabetes cannot be controlled with insulin. The limited supply of donor pancreases limits the number of transplants that can be done. According to Dr. Camillo Ricordi of the Diabetes Research Institute at the

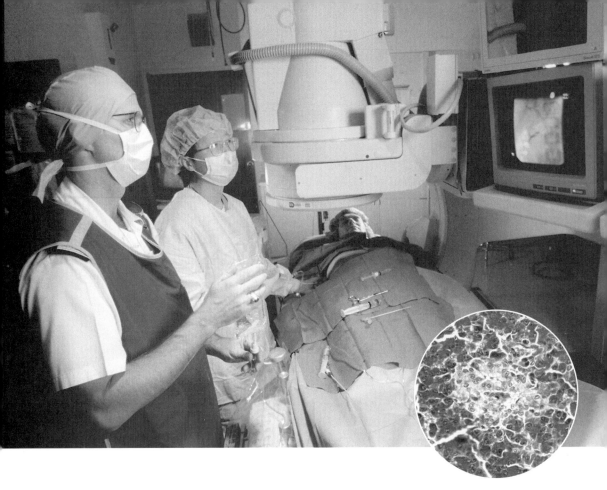

Surgeons transplant islets of Langerhans cells (inset) into a diabetic patient. This experimental procedure may lead to a cure for diabetes.

University of Miami, "Because we have only six thousand [dead] organ donors a year, there's no way we can fulfill the need for the millions that could benefit. And even if we could figure out a way to harvest cells from live donors, that's likely to only increase the number of transplants from a few thousand to tens of thousands."[53]

Success with Islet Transplantation

Islet transplantation is also receiving attention as a potential cure. Doctors have successfully extracted islets from donor pancreases and transplanted the cell clusters via a catheter into the liver. The liver is chosen as the transplant site because it is easy to place the islets next to the large vein of the liver, where they will have access to a blood supply.

In 1999 Canadian doctors transplanted islet cells into eight seriously ill patients with diabetes. They used a new combination of anti-rejection drugs and fresh, not previously frozen, islet cells. They also increased the number of transplanted islet cells to improve the chance a sufficient number of islet cells would survive the procedure. One year later, all eight patients were free of the need to take insulin injections.

Gary Kleiman is one of about a hundred diabetic patients in the United States who has received an islet transplant. Blind in one eye from diabetes and a survivor of two kidney transplants, Kleiman no longer needs the four to five insulin injections he used to take daily. About his islet cell transplant Kleiman said, "It's given my life a tremendous amount of freedom, flexibility, lack of worry and, in truth, it's given me a feeling of having a future."[54]

Unlike a pancreatic transplant, transplanting islets requires no major incisions. A catheter is used to put the cells in place and the patient remains awake under local anesthesia during surgery. However, the procedure is still experimental and there remain problems to solve.

Addressing Problems

A major problem with islet transplantation is the difficulty of harvesting sufficient islet cells and keeping the delicate tissues alive throughout the gathering and transplantation process. For an average-size person a total of about 1 million islets must be gathered, which typically consumes two donor pancreases. Since the number of donors is limited, researchers are experimenting with islet cells from pigs and genetically modified fish using immunosuppressive medications to prevent rejection. Scientists in California are also working to grow human beta cells in the laboratory.

To address the rejection problems associated with transplants of whole pancreases and islet cells, researchers have developed a hybrid artificial pancreas. Essentially the idea is to produce a protected islet transplant. Live islet cells are placed inside a tube or bag made of a membrane that exposes the islets to the blood stream but shields the islets from the body's immune response. The trick is in designing a membrane with holes too small for the islets to escape or the body's antibodies to enter. At the same time, the holes of the membrane need to be large enough for blood to flow through and carry off any insulin the islets produce in response to sugar in the blood. Keeping the cells alive is difficult. In addition, unlike the pancreas, hybrid artificial pancreases are not connected to the autonomic nervous system and thus are not cued to prepare insulin when chewing initiates the body's digestive cycle. Nonetheless, hybrid artificial pancreases have been successfully used in dogs, and human trials may begin shortly.

Changing immune markers could be another way to counter the rejection of transplanted organs or islet cells. According to Dr. Luca Inverardi, co-director of the cell transplant center at the Diabetes Research Institute, "Our major problem right now is that we have to give powerful generalized immunosuppression. . . . [This problem could be solved] if you could reeducate the immune system not to reject the transplanted organ, without compromising its ability to defend itself."[55]

Bone Marrow and Stem Cells

Bone marrow transplants might help address the issue of immune markers. From experience with cancer patients, doctors know transplanted bone marrow can exist alongside a patient's own bone marrow, giving the patient access to two immune systems. This arrangement allows the patient's body to accept cells or organs from the bone marrow donor. However, bone marrow transplants designed to give a patient access to two immune systems are still experimental at this time.

Researchers are also interested in bone marrow for another reason. Bone marrow contains stem cells, and stem cells have the potential to develop into any cell of the body. Researchers are exploring the possibility of using a person's own stem cells as a source of new beta cells. Research into the use of embryonic stem cells

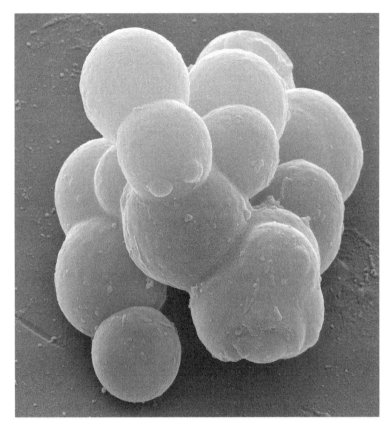

Stem cells can develop into any type of cell needed by the body. Researchers are exploring the use of stem cells as a cure for diabetes.

for the same purpose is also under way. Dr. Juan Dominguez Bendala at the Diabetes Research Institute in Miami says, "I think it's actually quite possible that we'll be using human embryonic stem cells to treat type 1 diabetes in the very near future."[56]

Genetic Interventions

Another approach to finding a cure for diabetes is gene therapy. Since diabetes—especially type 2 diabetes—is more common among people who have one or more family members with the disease, scientists continue to look for genetic causes or triggers of the disease. At this point, several genes have been uncovered and National Institutes of Health is funding research to discover all the genes that can influence the likelihood of a person getting diabetes. If the function of the various genes can be determined and scientists can identify changes that lead to diabetes, it may be possible to develop new treatments and perhaps even a cure.

In the meantime, researchers are looking into using genetic engineering techniques to insert the genetic code for producing insulin into the fat or muscle cells of a person with diabetes, thus creating a new set of cells that can produce insulin. However, there are still multiple questions that need to be resolved before this is feasible, including how the genetic code should be inserted, which cells the code should be inserted into, and how production of insulin will be regulated.

Another possibility would be to trigger the pancreas to make more insulin-producing cells. This might mean activating the same internal mechanism that creates more insulin-producing cells when a person gains weight. Another avenue might be to use chemical or hormonal prompts to encourage any remaining beta cells within the islets of Langerhans to reproduce and multiply.

Prevention

Perhaps the closest thing to a cure available today is prevention. New cases of type 2 diabetes are most common in people who are overweight and inactive. The muscle cells of overweight people seem to be less responsive to insulin. Frequently, there is a period when the pancreas produces more insulin to compensate for the body's resistance to insulin, but gradually the pancreas can no longer keep up. It loses more and more of its ability to produce insulin, leading to a shortage of insulin and the symptoms of diabetes. If a person loses weight, the production of insulin is sometimes sufficient to again maintain normal blood sugar levels.

In fact, research has shown maintaining normal weight and moderate exercise reduces the risk of getting type 2 diabetes. The Diabetes Prevention Program, a large prevention study of people at high risk for diabetes, found a 58 percent decrease in diabetes over three

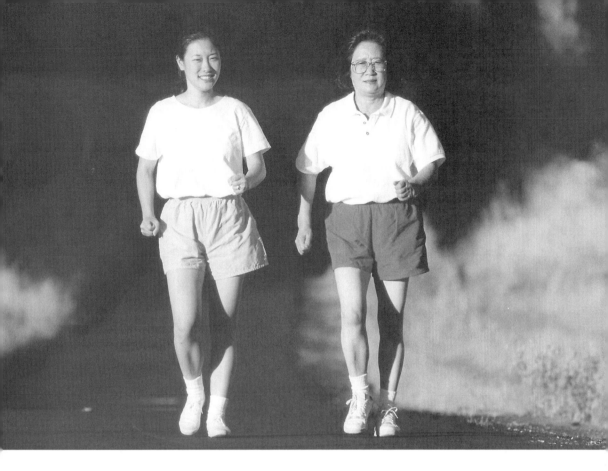

years among people who followed the healthy diet set forth by the program and exercised moderately. In other words, type 2 diabetes can be prevented or delayed in people at risk for diabetes. Losing 5 to 7 percent of body weight and exercising thirty minutes most days were enough to prevent or delay diabetes in the high-risk individuals studied. As a result, experts are doing their best to get the word out and encourage people to maintain a normal weight and exercise to prevent diabetes.

Preventing type 1 diabetes is less straightforward. Type 1 diabetes seems to occur when a person susceptible to diabetes produces an immune response that damages or destroys the beta cells of the islets. Scientists are looking at infections from viruses like Coxsackie B. The thought is that the immune system develops antibodies to fight the viral infection, but in susceptible individuals the antibodies also attack the beta cells because a protein on the cell surface is chemically similar to the virus.

Type 2 diabetes most often occurs in overweight, inactive people. Studies have shown that exercise and a healthy diet can prevent or delay diabetes.

In the meantime, an antibody named anti-CD3 has shown promise. When given to patients recently diagnosed with type 1 diabetes, anti-CD3 seemed to block the further destruction of the beta cells. Jeffery Bluestone, who developed the antibody, says, "Our animal research suggests that [the antibody] reorients the immune response. . . . in fact, the antibody may selectively inhibit previously activated immune cells that are involved in the development of diabetes."[57]

Dr. Kevan Herold of Columbia University, who conducted a clinical trial of anti-CD3 in humans, said, "The goal of this trial was to induce tolerance to the beta cell, which is the target of autoimmune destruction in type 1 diabetes. This was in effect achieved, because the clinical effect we saw persisted long after patients had finished treatment with the anti-CD3 antibody."[58] Indeed, patients participating in this trial who took anti-CD3 for fourteen days produced more insulin and needed less insulin therapy one year later than patients who did not receive the drug. Larger clinical trials are now being conducted with anti-CD3 to explore the potential of this antibody therapy as a possible cure for diabetes.

In looking at the broad picture, Dr. Camillo Ricordi notes, "There has been more progress in the last four years than the preceding two decades. But it's not a final victory."[59] Nevertheless, the hope for a cure for diabetes grows ever brighter.

NOTES

Introduction: Diabetes and the Miracle of Insulin

1. Quoted in Michael Bliss, *The Discovery of Insulin.* Chicago: University of Chicago Press, 1982, p. 22.
2. Frank N. Allan, "Diabetes Before and After Insulin," *Medical History*, July 1972, p. 272.
3. Quoted in Chris Feudtner, *Bittersweet: Diabetes, Insulin, and the Transformation of Illness.* Chapel Hill: University of North Carolina Press, 2003, p. 54.

Chapter 1: Treating the Sugar Sickness

4. Quoted in Jürgen Thorwald, translated by Richard and Clara Winston, *Science and Secrets of Early Medicine: Egypt, Mesopotamia, India, China, Mexico, Peru.* New York: Harcourt, Brace & World, 1962, p. 205.
5. Quoted in Joseph H. Barach, "Historical Facts in Diabetes," *Annals of Medical History*, vol. 10, 1928, p. 391.
6. Quoted in Barach, "Historical Facts in Diabetes," p. 390.
7. Quoted in Barach, "Historical Facts in Diabetes," p. 391.
8. Quoted in Bliss, *The Discovery of Insulin*, p. 23.
9. Quoted in Bliss, *The Discovery of Insulin*, p. 23.
10. Quoted in D.A. Pyke, "The History of Diabetes," p. 5. www.diabetesliving.com/basics/wiley.htm.

Chapter 2: Searching for a Cure

11. Quoted in Bliss, *The Discovery of Insulin*, p. 29.

12. Quoted in Bliss, *The Discovery of Insulin*, p. 30.
13. Quoted in Bliss, *The Discovery of Insulin*, p. 30.
14. Bliss, *The Discovery of Insulin*, p. 31.
15. Quoted in Aleita Hopping Scott, *Great Scott: Ernest Lyman Scott's Work with Insulin in 1911*. Bogota, NJ: Scott, 1972, p. 111.
16. Quoted in Scott, *Great Scott*, p. 113.
17. Ernest Lyman Scott, "On the Influence of Intravenous Injections of an Extract of the Pancreas on Experimental Pancreatic Diabetes," *American Journal of Physiology*, January 1, 1912, p. 310.
18. Quoted in Scott, *Great Scott*, p. 123.

Chapter 3: The Summer and Fall of 1921

19. Quoted in Bliss, *The Discovery of Insulin*, pp. 49–50.
20. Quoted in Bliss, *The Discovery of Insulin*, p. 53.
21. Quoted in Henry B.M. Best, *Margaret and Charley: The Personal Story of Dr. Charles Best, the Co-Discoverer of Insulin*. Toronto: Dundurn Group, 2003, p. 47.
22. Quoted in Best, *Margaret and Charley*, p. 51.
23. C.H. Best, "Reminiscences of the Researches Which Led to the Discovery of Insulin," *Canadian Medical Association Journal*, November 1942, p. 400.
24. Quoted in Bliss, *The Discovery of Insulin*, p. 67.
25. F.G. Banting and C.H. Best, "The Internal Secretion of the Pancreas," *Journal of Laboratory and Clinical Medicine*, February 1922, p. 254.
26. Quoted in Bliss, *The Discovery of Insulin*, p. 70.
27. Quoted in Bliss, *The Discovery of Insulin*, p. 73.
28. Quoted in Best, *Margaret and Charley*, p. 54.
29. Ffrangcon Roberts, "Insulin" Correspondence, *British Medical Journal*, December 16, 1922, p. 1194.
30. Quoted in Bliss, *The Discovery of Insulin*, p. 109.

Chapter 4: Behind the Scenes

31. Quoted in Best, *Margaret and Charley*, p. 56.
32. Quoted in Bliss, *The Discovery of Insulin*, p. 104.
33. Quoted in Best, *Margaret and Charley*, p. 62.

34. Quoted in Bliss, *The Discovery of Insulin*, p. 107.
35. Charles H. Best, "Reminiscences of the Discovery of Insulin: The First Clinical Use of Insulin," *Diabetes*, January–February 1956, p. 66.
36. Quoted in Bliss, *The Discovery of Insulin*, p. 117.
37. Quoted in Bliss, *The Discovery of Insulin*, p. 118.
38. Quoted in Best, *Margaret and Charley*, p. 64.
39. Quoted in Paul de Kruif, *Men Against Death*. New York: Harcourt, Brace, 1932, p. 81.
40. Quoted in Bliss, *The Discovery of Insulin*, p. 127.
41. Quoted in Best, *Margaret and Charley*, p. 66.
42. Quoted in Bliss, *The Discovery of Insulin*, p. 134.
43. de Kruif, *Men Against Death*, pp. 83–84.
44. Pyke, "The History of Diabetes," p. 5.
45. Quoted in Bliss, *The Discovery of Insulin*, p. 172.

Chapter 5: Insulin and Technology Today

46. Allan, "Diabetes Before and After Insulin," p. 267.
47. Bliss, *The Discovery of Insulin*, p. 245.
48. David Bjerklie, "The Other Diabetes," *Time*, November 30, 2003. www.drinet.org/html/november_30__2003.htm.
49. Quoted in Carol Lewis, "Diabetes: A Growing Public Health Concern," *FDA Consumer Magazine*, January–February 2002, p. 5. www.fda.gov/fdac/features/2002/102_diab.html.
50. Quoted in Maria Collazo-Clavell, *Mayo Clinic on Managing Diabetes*. Rochester, MN: Mayo Foundation for Medical Education and Research, 2001, p. 39.

Chapter 6: Future Hopes for a Cure

51. Richard Beaser and Joan V.C. Hill, *The Joslin Guide to Diabetes: A Program for Managing Your Treatment*. New York: Simon & Schuster, 1995, pp. 109–110.
52. Quoted in Lewis, "Diabetes: A Growing Public Health Concern," p. 6.
53. Quoted in Bjerklie, "The Other Diabetes."
54. Quoted in "University of Miami Leading the Way in Fight Against Diabetes," NBC6.net, January 5, 2004, p. 2. www.nbc6.net/health/2742722/detail.htm.

55. Quoted in Daniela Lamas, "Transplant Gives Patient a Future," *Miami Herald*, February 10, 2004, p. 2. www.drinet.org/html/february_10__2004.htm.

56. Robert Bazell, "The Limits of Stem Cells: Current Research Unlikely to Benefit Patients with Alzheimer's Disease," *The Nightly News with Tom Brokaw*, July 27, 2004, p. 1. www.drinet.org/html/july_2004.htm.

57. Quoted in National Institute of Diabetes & Digestive & Kidney Diseases, "Studies Yield Key Insights in Preventing Destruction of Insulin-Producing Cells," May 29, 2002, p. 2. www.niddk.nih.gov/welcome/releases/05-29-02.htm.

58. National Institute of Diabetes & Digestive & Kidney Diseases, "Studies Yield Key Insights," p. 2.

59. Quoted in Daniela Lamas, "Transplant Gives Patient a Future," p. 2.

FOR FURTHER READING

Books

American Diabetes Association, *American Diabetes Association Complete Guide to Diabetes.* Alexandria, VA: American Diabetes Association, 1996. A straightforward presentation of the causes and symptoms of diabetes and how to manage the disease, including types of insulin, oral medications, diet, exercise, complications, and available tools and technology.

Alden R. Carter, *I'm Tougher than Diabetes!* Morton Grove, IL: Albert Whitman, 2001. Informally told and full of photos, this is a book in which a young girl with type 1 diabetes shares her life, including how she tracks her blood sugar and copes with the disease.

Seale Harris, *Banting's Miracle: The Story of the Discoverer of Insulin,* Philadelphia: J.B. Lippincott, 1946. A highly readable biography of Frederick Banting's life, including his discovery of insulin.

Web Sites

American Diabetes Association (www.diabetes.org/about-diabetes.jsp). The American Diabetes Association funds research, publishes scientific findings, and provides information on diabetes to the public and health professionals. The Web site contains general information on diabetes as well as information on specific topics related to treatment and better understanding of the disease. The language can be a little technical, but the site contains lots of brief descriptions of topics related to diabetes.

Children with Diabetes (www.childrenwithdiabetes. com/sitemap/htm). An online organization for children with diabetes and their parents. In addition to general information on diabetes, the site is full of practical information on how to cope with diabetes. It includes information on related events and has a list of teens and preteens with diabetes who want to talk with each other and share experiences. There is an opportunity to ask health professionals specific questions about diabetes.

National Diabetes Information Clearinghouse (http:// diabetes.niddk.nih.gov). A clearinghouse for diabetes information, the Web site contains general information on diabetes, specific information on diabetes-related topics, and links to other organizations with information on diabetes.

University of Toronto Libraries, Fisher Library Digital Collections (http://digital.library.utoronto.ca/insulin). A veritable gold mine, this Web site contains over seven thousand images from the collections of Fred Banting, Charles Best, and others related to the discovery of insulin that are housed at the University of Toronto Libraries. The material covers the time period from 1920 to 1925 and includes images of original laboratory notebooks, letters from patients, photographs, awards, newspaper clippings, and Banting's personal scrapbook. Also included are biographies of Banting, Best, James Collip, and J.J.R. Macleod and related information on the discovery of insulin.

WORKS CONSULTED

Books

Richard Beaser and Joan V.C. Hill, *"The Joslin Guide to Diabetes: A Program for Managing Your Treatment.* New York: Simon & Schuster, 1995. Written to help people with diabetes understand the disease and how to manage it, this book discusses both the disease and how to live with it. The book uses technical and medical terms but defines them as they are introduced so the reader can understand the content as it is presented.

Henry B.M. Best, *Margaret and Charley: The Personal Story of Dr. Charles Best, the Co-Discover of Insulin.* Toronto: Dundurn Group, 2003. Written by Charles H. Best's son, this book tells the story of Charles Best and his wife, Margaret Mahon Best. Based on Margaret's journals and Charley's letters, it tells the story not only of the discovery of insulin but of the life and work of this remarkable couple.

Michael Bliss, *The Discovery of Insulin.* Chicago: University of Chicago Press, 1982. Written by a historian, this book contains an extensively researched but easy-to-follow history of the discovery of insulin. Drawn from the original lab books, personal notes, correspondence, and the scientific literature, it weaves together the context, events, and personalities involved in the discovery of insulin.

Jennie Brand-Miller, Kaye Foster-Powell, and Rick Mendosa, *What Makes My Blood Glucose Go Up ... and Down? And 101 Other Frequently Asked Questions About Your Blood Glucose Levels.* New York: Marlowe, 2003. This book answers frequently asked questions about blood glucose levels and how food, exercise, mood, and stress affect those levels. Written in a casual, sometimes funny style, it defines many scientific and medical terms and includes a glossary.

Maria Collazo-Clavell, *Mayo Clinic on Managing Diabetes.* Rochester, MN: Mayo Foundation for Medical Education and Research, 2001. This easy-to-read book provides an overview of diabetes and how to manage the disease, including medications available, types of insulin, new technologies, and hopes for a cure. Includes diagrams to help further understand the material presented.

Chris Feudtner, *Bittersweet: Diabetes, Insulin, and the Transformation of Illness*. Chapel Hill: University of North Carolina Press, 2003. This book is based on detailed patient records kept by Dr. Elliott P. Joslin over his sixty years of treating people with diabetes, both before and after the discovery of insulin. Feudtner looks at the transformation of diabetes from a deadly to a chronic disease, with an emphasis on how coping with the chronic aspects and complications of diabetes affects people with diabetes and their loved ones.

Helen V. Fisher, *Type II Diabetes and Your Health*. Tucson, AZ: Fisher, 2000. Although this work is primarily a cookbook, the first thirty pages offer an overview of the different types of diabetes. Fisher emphasizes the symptoms and complications of type 2 diabetes, including medications available and how to manage type 2 diabetes through diet and exercise.

Folke Henschen, translated by Joan Tate, *The History of Diseases*. London: Longmans, Green, 1966. A review of the geographic and historical distribution of diseases throughout the world. Fairly technical language with photos and illustrations of diseases throughout history.

Paul de Kruif, *Men Against Death*. New York: Harcourt, Brace, 1932. Based on a review of the scientific literature and personal interviews with nine of the twelve discoverers profiled, this book tells the stories of great medical discoveries and their discoverers. Written in 1932, the stories are told in a romantic and flowery style that is enjoyable to read.

Marvin E. Levin and Michael A. Pfeifer, eds., *The Uncomplicated Guide to Diabetes Complications*. Alexandria, VA: American Diabetes Association, 2002. Organized into chapters by type of complication, the book provides a clear discussion of the common complications of diabetes, what can be done to prevent each complication, and how to recognize and treat the symptoms. Includes stories of people who are coping with complications of diabetes.

Annette Maggi and Jackie Boucher, *What You Can Do to Prevent Diabetes: Simple Changes to Improve Your Life*. New York: John Wiley, 2000. Written with short chapters, this book focuses on preventing diabetes through good nutrition and exercise. It provides readers the tools and motivation to change their lifestyle.

Stanley Mirsky and Joan Rattner Heilman, *Controlling Diabetes the Easy Way*. New York: Random House, 1998. An overview of diabetes designed to help people with diabetes understand and manage the disease.

Christopher D. Saudek, Richard R. Rubin, and Cynthia S. Shump, *The Johns Hopkins Guide to Diabetes for Today and Tomorrow*. Baltimore: Johns Hopkins University Press, 1997. A comprehensive review of diabetes, including complications and treatment, this book features quotes and stories from people with diabetes.

Aleita Hopping Scott, *Great Scott: Ernest Lyman Scott's Work with Insulin in 1911*. Bogota, NJ: Scott, 1972. The first half of this book written by Ernest Lyman Scott's wife consists of notes taken from an extended conversation with her husband about his extraction of insulin. The second half of the book provides a biography of Ernest Lyman Scott and his work to extract insulin from the pancreas.

Jürgen Thorwald, translated by Richard and Clara Winston, *Science and Secrets of Early Medicine: Egypt, Mesopotamia, India, China, Mexico, Peru*. New York: Harcourt, Brace & World, 1962. A review of the history, illnesses, and medical knowledge of early civilizations. Contains hundreds of photos and drawings of mummies, ancient writings, figurines and sculptures, and medical illustrations and art, all related to disease and medicine among early peoples.

Periodicals and Reports

Frank N. Allan, "Diabetes Before and After Insulin," *Medical History*, July 1972.

F.G. Banting and C.H. Best, "The Internal Secretion of the Pancreas," *Journal of Laboratory and Clinical Medicine*, February 1922.

F. G Banting, C.H. Best, J.B. Collip, W.R. Campbell, and A.A. Fletcher, "Pancreatic Extracts in the Treatment of Diabetes Mellitus," an abridgment from the *Canadian Medical Association Journal*, March 1922, *Diabetes*, January–February 1956.

W.M. Bayliss, "Insulin, Diabetes, and Rewards for Discoveries," *Nature*, February 10, 1923.

Charles H. Best, "The History of Insulin," *Diabetes*, November–December 1962.

———, "Reminiscences of the Discovery of Insulin: The First Clinical Use of Insulin," *Diabetes*, January–February 1956.

———, "Reminiscences of the Researches Which Led to the Discovery of Insulin," *Canadian Medical Association Journal*, November 1942.

Joseph H. Barach, "Historical Facts in Diabetes," *Annals of Medical History*, vol. 10, 1928.

H.I. Burtness and E.F. Cain, "A Thirty-fifth Anniversary of Insulin Therapy and a Sixty-fifth Wedding Anniversary," *Diabetes*, January–February 1958.

Robert Cooke, "Medicine Awaiting a Diabetes Breakthrough," *Newsday*, September 2, 1986.

H.H. Dale, "Insulin" Correspondence, *British Medical Journal*, December 23, 1922.

Victoria Stagg Elliott, "Scientists Strive to Spare Diabetics from the Needle," *American Medical News*, September 17, 2001.

Janet Enright, "Parents Struggle to Cope with Their Children's Diabetes," *Toronto Star*, October 11, 1988.

John F. Fulton, "Reminiscences of the Discovery of Insulin: Sir Frederick Banting 1891–1941," *Diabetes*, January–February 1956.

Penelope Johnson, "One Sleepless Night Makes History: Diabetes Treatment Theorized," *Medical Post*, February 6, 2001.

Elliott P. Joslin, "Reminiscences of the Discovery of Insulin: A Personal Impression," *Diabetes*, January–February 1956.

O. Leyton, "Treatment of Diabetes Mellitus with Insulin," *The Lancet*, November 24, 1923.

Joan MacCracken and Donna Hoel, "From Ants to Analogues: Puzzles and Promises in Diabetes Management," *Postgraduate Medicine*, April 1997.

J.J.R. Macleod, "Insulin and Diabetes: A General Statement of the Physiological and Therapeutic Effects of Insulin," *British Medical Journal*, November 4, 1922.

Ian Murray, "Paulesco and the Isolation of Insulin," *Journal of the History of Medicine*, vol. XXVI (2), 1971.

———, "The Search for Insulin," *Scottish Medical Journal*, vol. 14, 1969.

"Pipeline Report: Insulin Options Are Coming—but Not Soon," *Washington Post*, August 21, 2001.

"The Preparation of Insulin," *British Medical Journal*, December 23, 1922.

Ffrangcon Roberts, "Insulin" Correspondence. *British Medical Journal*, December 16, 1922.

Ernest Lyman Scott, "The Effect of Pancreas Extract on Depancreatized Dogs: A Dissertation Submitted to the Faculty of the Ogden Graduate School of Science in Candidacy for the Degree of Masters of Science Department of Physiology," Thesis No. T-10553. Chicago: University of Chicago, Summer 1911.

———, "On the Influence of Intravenous Injections of an Extract of the Pancreas on Experimental Pancreatic Diabetes," *American Journal of Physiology*, January 1, 1912.

John L. Sievenpiper, Alexandra L. Jenkins, Dana L. Whitham, and Vladimir Vuksan, "Insulin Resistance: Concepts, Controversies, and the Role of Nutrition," *Canadian Journal of Dietetic Practice and Research*, vol. 63, no. 1, Spring 2002.

Stephen Smith, "Lab Cracks a Key Letter in Body's Insulin Code: Way Seen to Prod Cells of Diabetes," *Boston Globe*, August 6, 2002.

"The Treatment of Diabetes by Insulin," *British Medical Journal*, November 18, 1922.

Warren T. Vaughan, "The Diabetic Diet," *Journal of Laboratory and Clinical Medicine*, August 1922.

Internet Sources

American Diabetes Association, "Islet Replacement Research Awards," November 20, 2003. www.diabetes.org/diabetes-research/ADA-Research-Foundation/islet-cell-replacement-research-awards.jsp.

———, "National Diabetes Fact Sheet." www.diabetes.org/diabetes-statistics/national-diabetes-fact-sheet.jsp.

———, "Type 2 Diabetes Prevention Research Awards," November 4, 2003. www.diabetes.org/diabetes-research/ADA-Research-Foundation/type2-prevention-awards.jsp.

Robert Bazell, "The Limits of Stem Cells: Current Research Unlikely to Benefit Patients with Alzheimer's Disease," *The Nightly News with Tom Brokaw*, July 27, 2004. www.drinet.org/html/july_2004.htm.

Henry B.M. Best, "Speech to the Academy of Medicine," delivered at the Vaughan Estate in Toronto, April 24, 1996. www.discoveryofinsulin.com/Best.htm.

David Bjerklie, "The Other Diabetes," *Time*, November 30, 2003. www.drinet.org/html/november_30__2003.htm.

Canadian Medicine: Doctors and Discoveries, "A Great Canadian Breakthrough: The Discovery of Insulin," updated 2001. www.mta.ca/faculty/arts/canadian_5Fstudies/english/about/study_5guide/doctors/insulin.html.

Centers for Disease Control and Prevention, National Center for Chronic Disease Prevention and Health Promotion, "Diabetes: Frequently Asked Questions," updated June 17, 2004. www.cdc.gov/diabetes/faqs.htm.

———, "National Diabetes Fact Sheet," updated May 12, 2004. www.cdc.gov/diabetes/pubs/general.htm.

Children with Diabetes, "Insulin Pump Therapy," updated November 15, 2004. www.childrenwithdiabetes.com/pumps/.

———, "Pump Basics," updated May 12, 2004. www.childrenwithdiabetes.com/pumps.basics.htm.

Manuel Luciano da Silva, "Diabetes Means Siphon! Insulin Comes from the Islands." www.apol.net/dightonrock/diabetes_history.htm.

Michael Dick, "The Ancient Ayurvedic Writings." www.ayurveda.com/online%20resource/ancient_writings.htm.

Discovery of Insulin, "A Brief Biography of Dr. F.G. Banting." www.discoveryofinsulin.com/Banting.htm.

———, "Biography: Charles Herbert Best." www.discoveryofinsulin.com/Best.htm.

———, "Biography: James Bertram Collip." www.discoveryofinsulin.com/Collip.htm.

———, "Biography: John James Rickard Macleod." www.discoveryofinsulin.com/Macleod.htm.

———, "The History of Diabetes Treatment," updated 2003. www.inventors.about.com/library/inventors/bldiabetes.htm.

———, "Insulin: A Canadian Medical Miracle of the 20th Century." www.discoveryofinsulin.com/Introduction.htm.

Encyclopedia Britannica Online, "DeWitt, Lydia Maria Adams." www.britannica.com/eb/article?tocID=9030191.

Shane T. Grey, "Genetic Engineering and Xenotransplantation," May 2000. www.actionbioscience.org/biotech/grey.html.

Health Central—General Encyclopedia, "Diabetes Mellitus." www.healthcentral.com/mhc/top/001214.cfm.

Insulin-Free World, "Facts and Statistics," www.insulin-free.org/factspan.html.

International Pancreas Transplant Registry, "International Pancreas Transplant Registry Midyear Update 2003," www.iptr.umn.edu/ar_midyear2003/03_midyear_ update_page_1.htm.

Nan C. Jensen, "Diabetes." http://coopo.co.pinellas.fl.us/TimeTweb/2001/march01/marnan.htm.

KidsHealth, "The Real Deal on the Digestive System," March 2004. http://kidshealth.org/kid/body/digest_noSW.html.

Daniela Lamas, "Cell Transplant Gives Patient a Future," *Miami Herald*, February 10, 2004. www.drinet.org/html/february_10__2004.htm.

Lemelson–MIT Program, "Inventor of the Week: Helen Free," updated February 1999. http://web.mit.edu/invent/iow/free.html.

Carol Lewis, "Diabetes: A Growing Public Health Concern," *FDA Consumer Magazine*, January–February 2002. www.fda.gov/fdac/features/2002/102_diab.html.

"Life with Diabetes." www.lifewithdiabetes.co.uk/page25.html.

J.J.R. Macleod, "Nobel Speech: The Physiology of Insulin and Its Source in the Animal Body," Nobel lecture delivered in Stockholm, Sweden, on May 26, 1925. www.discoveryofinsulin.com/Macleod.htm.

National Institute of Diabetes & Digestive & Kidney Diseases, "Alternative Devices for Taking Insulin," updated August 2004. www.niddk.nih.gov/dm/pubs/insulin/index.htm.

————, "Noninvasive Blood Glucose Monitors," updated October 2003. www.niddk.nih.gov/dm/pubs/glucosemonitor/index. htm.

————, "Pancreatic Islet Transplantation," updated November 2003. www.niddk.nih.gov/dm/pubs/pancreaticislet/index.htm.

————, "Studies Yield Key Insights in Preventing Destruction of Insulin-Producing Cells," May 29, 2002. www.niddk.nih.gov/ welcome/releases/05-29-02.htm.

National Inventors Hall of Fame, "Helen Free." www.invent. org/hall_of_fame/63.html.

National Women's Health Information Center, "Diabetes: Overview," updated March 2003. www.4woman.gov/faq/diabetes.htm.

NBC6.net, "University of Miami Leading the Way in Fight Against Diabetes," January 5, 2004. www.nbc6.net/health/2742722/ detail.htm.

Neurology Channel, "Coma: Overview," updated March 9, 2004. http://neurologychannel.com/coma.

Nigel Phillips, "Brunner, Johann Conrad," in Bibliopoly. www. polybiblio.com/phillips/368.html.

Novo Nordisk Ireland, "History of Diabetes." www.novonordisk. ie/view.asp?ID=1200.

Public Broadcasting Service, "A Science Odyssey: People and Discoveries: Banting and Best Isolate Insulin, 1922." www. pbs.org/wgbh/aso/databank/entries/dm22in.html.

D.A. Pyke, "The History of Diabetes." www.diabetesliving.com/ basics/wiley.htm.

Brandon Reines, "The Truth Behind the Discovery of Insulin." www.animalvoices.org/insulin1.htm.

Sugar India, "Diabetes Timeline." www.sugarindia.com/diabtime. htm.

Vanesa Sutherland, "Glossary of Terms." www.insulin-free.org/ glossary.htm.

INDEX

Picture Credits

About the Author

Janice M. Yuwiler has her master's degree in public health and has spent over fifteen years working with health organizations to prevent children and adolescents from being injured. She has a background in epidemiology and molecular biology and delights in putting the latest break-throughs in science and medicine in the hands of young people. Her other book published with Lucent Books is *Family Violence*. Yuwiler is a native Californian who enjoys living in sunny California with her husband and three children.